CHRONICLES OF THE CHRISTMAS REINDEER

WAYNE H. BOMAR

Dragonfire
Productions

Copyright © 1996 by Wayne H. (Bo) Bomar. All rights reserved.

Edited by:
Isabel Anders

Cover by:
Charles Hooper, Nashville, TN

Back cover photo by:
Dan Loftin

Design, typography, and text production by:
Christine Shook, TypeByte Graphix

ISBN: 1-886371-51-2

Dragonfire Productions
145 Bledsoe Park Road
Gallatin, TN 37066
1-615-452-1028

For ordering information 1-800-396-4626

To Santa and Mrs. Claus... It was your dream that the love of the Christmas Reindeer be shared with the entire world.

To my wife, Elaine... You helped me find the magic again. You are truly the ninth-chosen Christmas Reindeer; and together we shall travel the magical winds of Christmas forever. I love you!

To Mama and Daddy, Mary Sue Bomar and Joseph Comar Bomar... Your love and belief in me are intertwined within the pages of this book. I'll remember, Pop!

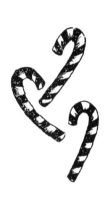

To Joe and Linda Tatar... What can I say? You believed in me.

To the children of the world, old and young alike.

And especially to Donder, my friend... You found me when I was alone. You drew the curtains back and let the magic shine in. You gave me all that you possessed and more. You are with me always, my brother. May the eternal winds of Christmas always be at your back... your course clear. I shall remember and believe... forever believe!

Contents

Acknowledgments	vii
Introduction	ix
1. The Journey Begins—Christmas Eve Magic	1
2. Cupid's Dilemma	13
3. A High-Climb Run and Grandfather Blitzen	21
4. A Christmas Gift for Grandfather Blitzen	31
5. Children of the Reindeer and Thoughts of Home	41
6. An Emergency of Highest Priority	51
7. A Homecoming for Dancer and Prancer	61
8. A Christmas Eve Party—North Pole Style	73
9. Christmas Magic and Donder's Story	83
10. Christmas Breakfast with Santa and Blitzen's Story of Love	95
11. A Visit with Santa and a Ride with Comet	109
12. A Visit with Vixen and the Valley of Christmas Trees	119
13. The Littlest Christmas Reindeer	129
14. Santa's Christmas Assignments and Vixen's Workroom	139
15. The Christmas Jobs of Dasher and Comet	149
16. An Evening at Grandfather Blitzen's	161
17. A Christmas Reindeer Named Vixen	171
18. A Trip to Iceland	181
19. Dasher's Birthday and His Great Speed	189
20. Dasher's Magical Story	199
21. A Get-Together at Cupid's	209
22. Comet: Brother of the Wind	219
23. Dancer and Prancer: A Tale of Great Reindeer	229
24. Never Say Good-Bye	241
25. With Love, From All of Us	249

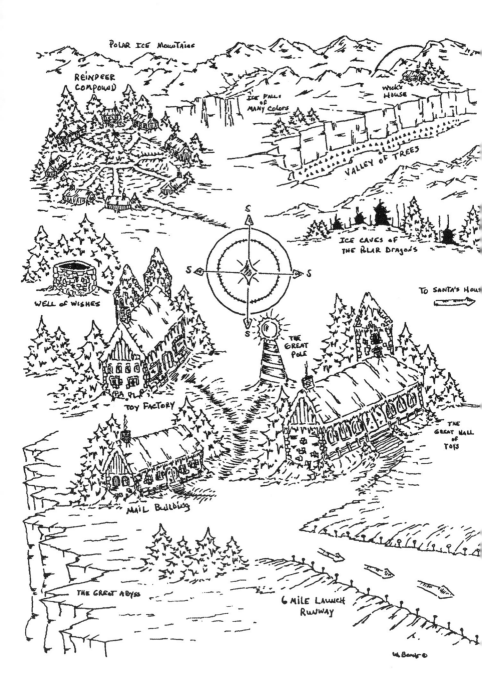

Acknowledgments

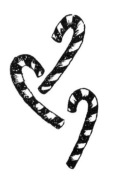

With all my heart I wish to thank:

Grandfather Blitzen,

Donder,

Dasher,

Dancer,

Prancer,

Comet,

Vixen,

and

little Cupid.

What a wondrous gift you all are.

Introduction

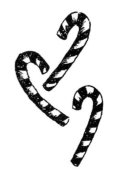

> *"In the magical land of ice and snow where the good Santa Claus covers the ice mountains with his booming laughter, there is peace, love, and happiness."*
> —*Donder, 1989 A.D.*

I have seen it! It is there! *They* are there—all of them! The eight Christmas Reindeer of love. Such wonders you cannot imagine. They chose me to write their adventures down as they have lived and continue to live.

In this book you will hear the exciting stories of Santa's eight Reindeer. Their adventures are an ongoing wonder. As long as there is but one smile on a child's face, they will continue to live.

Grandfather Blitzen told me on a cold, clear night one November: "Be kind, be gentle. Cherish the children, for they are love in its purest form. Revel in their laughter, their touch, and their smiles. They believe in the magic of goodness. Everyone can learn from the innocence of children. If we could be as the children are and see the goodness in everything... aye, what a magnificent world this would be."

Let me share with you these wonderful Christmas Reindeer: the secret of their origins; who and *why* they are what they are; their closeness to each other and their unbounded love for the children of the entire world. For over 1,700 years they have danced on the winds of Christmas Eve magic: Blitzen, Donder, Dasher, Dancer, Prancer, Comet, Vixen, and little Cupid. Their stories are all here... for you.

Lad

> "If 'tis a smile ye seek, give a gift; if 'tis love and happiness ye seek, give of yourself."
> —Grandfather Blitzen, 1301 A.D.

> "Don't be afraid to believe. Follow your own heart, for therein lies the truth of your own self."
> —Dasher, 1971 A.D.

> "In a sense, they are not my Reindeer. They belong to the children of the entire world. They belong to the young at heart. They love you... all of you."
> —Santa Claus, 1996 A.D.

1

The Journey Begins—Christmas Eve Magic

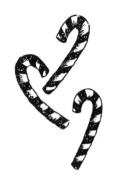

Christmas Eve, 1968... and now, as I write, I cannot remember ever feeling as sad as I did on that night. It was partly the time of the year, and I do remember thinking, *Why me?* My car was not running. I was out of money. It was raining a cold drizzle and I was on foot—having left my transportation some three miles behind me. I was headed for home.

It was a home that housed no Christmas tree, no decorations, no presents. I remember I was crying. Pretty childish for a man of forty. I remember thinking of Christmases past when I had been happy: A family, childhood fantasies come true, Christmas trees, many decorations. But then, I had grown up, entered the "real" world, as so many people call it. Now I felt that it was sometimes an ugly place, this real world. *What had happened to the Christmas of my childhood?*

Even at that low point, I wanted to believe in what reality said I couldn't. I must have walked crying in that cold rain for hours, feeling sorry for myself, telling myself that life wasn't worth this. It was freezing, and I had no more bright outlooks—nothing really to hope for.

That's when I heard the sound. I will always call it "the sound" though that hardly describes what I heard. I was miles from a city. I lived in an old farmhouse. The woods around me were dark, wet, gloomy, and cold. Startled, I looked quickly up when I heard the sound. I should have been the only one for miles around. Yet what was this? It was like tinkling glass or tiny bells hitting against each other. An almost musical sound.

Although it was many years ago, I still remember the first time I heard that sound. I saw nothing as I scanned the open fields and woods around me. *My mind must be playing tricks on me again,* I thought. I continued to walk through the cold drizzle—and then I heard the sound again. Looking up quickly, I saw a flash of light. Nothing big or spectacular. More like the beam of a pen flashlight. And yet, it reminded me of something—something long ago. It was like a flash of candlelight through a crack in the curtains, or the way icicles gleam when the sun hits them. *The fear I had felt was gone.*

I was filled with something else. Security? Or maybe it was a sense of not being alone. I felt as though someone was protecting me, watching over me. It was a good feeling, a sense of being *loved.*

I had a new appreciation of life around me. Even in that cold drizzle and grayness, I suddenly felt warm. The sound and light came again, but this time much closer. The sweet tinkling of bells, a flash of brilliant silver—with which the sun could not compare itself.

A quiet sense of joy filled me, and I couldn't help remembering the book *A Christmas Carol* by Charles Dickens.

The darkness wasn't there anymore. I was surrounded by the most brilliant light I had ever encountered. The bells were louder, and I could hear footsteps. They weren't loud, but they gave the impression that the person making them was very large indeed.

As I looked, a shape began moving toward me—quickly, but with deliberate cause. Yet I felt no fear, no panic. I think I even amazed myself with my own steadiness.

Then, as the shape neared me, I heard the boom of laughter. Yet it was a peaceful laughter, unlike anything I had ever heard. When I looked up—it wasn't a shape before me, it was a person. And he was dressed in brilliant red—in fact, a more brilliant red has not been made. A robe of red flowed just above the cold ground, and he was supported by the blackest boots I had ever seen. They were laced-up boots and, curiously, they had shiny specks covering the lower heels. These specks were of silver and gold and every color known to humans—and maybe some that weren't.

In my childhood dreams of long ago, I had imagined that this person would look like this. His hands were on his hips, and he was looking down at me and chuckling. He was enormous—not just in girth, but also in height. He was at least two feet taller than I was—and I guess I'm about average height. As he looked at me, there in the cold drizzle, I felt maybe I had died. What one wishes for all his life cannot suddenly appear. Reality had taught me that.

And yet..., he was very old, it seemed. His whiskers were the whitest color imaginable, and the hat on his head was the same brilliant red as his suit, with a single bell fastened to the long tassel that hung to his shoulders. A white material trimmed his clothes with the shiny luster of silk. I was unaware of everything around me except him. He filled the woods, the sky, the meadows. He was a part of the landscape. I couldn't take my eyes off him.

"Well, Lad, tell me what you think," he said, still chuckling. What could anyone say? I couldn't think. I opened my mouth to speak, but the only word that came out was *"Santa."* Again, his booming laughter hit my ears.

"We have a story to tell, Lad, and you're the one to tell it," he said. "If you've no objection, I would like you to come with us and write the story. You're a writer. Maybe just a little down on your luck right now—but nevertheless, a writer with great feeling. We choose you to tell our story to; and you in turn will tell it to the world!"

He talked in the plural, of "we." Yet I could see only him. What had he meant? As if reading my thoughts, he turned, and, with a wave of his arm, revealed a storybook tale come true. I saw the sleigh, the Reindeer, the bells, the presents, the shiny specks covering everything. And it had started to snow.

I suddenly began to cry. Yet it was a cry of joy and warmth and great emotion over *all that I had forgotten about as I had grown up. They were here in front of me.* Not in a book or a movie. *Right here.* As real as the trees around me and the soft, white snow falling on my head. I was filled with Christmas, with make-believe, with happiness and love. I was overcome by a love so big that words cannot do it justice.

I was meeting Santa Claus! As a child I remember calling for him, pleading with him to take me with him so that I might become a part of something I loved so much. And now my wish had come true.

"We must hurry, Lad. There's much to do tonight, and you have your work cut out for you. Your writing pads and pens are in the sleigh. You must record everything you see and hear, for tonight is a magical night, and there will be much to tell."

He led me toward the sleigh and steered me to the front of the line of Reindeer. "Introductions are in order, Lad. You must know the ones you will write about, and they in turn must know you. It is their story—one that has been told only briefly in the past two hundred years or so. You will write about what they think and experience."

I cast aside my doubts—although later, I must confess, I realized that I never really *had* any doubts. I wanted to believe, and so I did. Before I met Santa and the Reindeer, my childhood had become buried beneath "reality." I had let go of the magic that had held me so securely as a child. But, in the twinkling of Santa's eye, that magic had returned a hundredfold!

Santa wanted me to write down the long-overdue life histories and adventures of the Christmas Reindeer! I sensed the Reindeers' intelligence, and the love that each felt for the man dressed in red. And despite all the stories that had been written about the man called "Santa Claus," they felt no envy or jealousy. Only love shone forth from their eyes. This was to be their Christmas present from Santa: The story of their lives, to be told to believers and nonbelievers alike.

It was their turn, Santa told me. "For centuries, they have pulled this sleigh, loaded with millions of Christmas presents for boys and girls from all over the world. They have never complained of the load or the weather, but have pulled earnestly in their traces so that Christmas magic might be spread over the world. They have seen difficult times and been burdened by heavy loads; but always their hearts were full. And they have always answered my calls with a twinkle in their eyes.

"Beasts of burden? No. Reindeer of love, with a mission as important as time itself in their very hearts and souls. They have never complained. The people must know of their stout hearts and strong backs that have never failed me or the children of the world every Christmas Eve. You will see their magic, Lad, and you will believe even more than you do now."

As we stood there in the falling snow, Santa Claus, the Reindeer, and I, he began to introduce them. As he called each name, I would feel the love pour forth and roll off his tongue. He briefly cupped each Reindeer's muzzle in his white gloves and scratched each one behind the ear.

"The lead Reindeer, always to the left, is Blitzen. He is the oldest of my Reindeer. He knows the wind-currents of a thousand years and can follow the true path my sleigh must take. The others follow Blitzen without question. You will hear the story of his noble life before long."

Later, Santa would tell me that although age was taking its toll on his oldest Reindeer, the others would never question a limp or a misplaced hoof if a rooftop landing should not be as graceful as the first. It was not unusual, he said, for the others to sneak extra food to Blitzen when they thought Santa's back was turned.

"Donder is beside Blitzen as second lead Reindeer in the traces," Santa continued. "He has remained so for nearly 1,200 mortal years. Donder is quick-a-foot and will take the lead when Blitzen occasionally naps —which is permitted from time to time. A stronger

Reindeer than Donder was never born, and he will pull his heart out if I let him."

Donder looked up at me and winked with the sparkle of stardust in his eyes. It was Donder that I would grow closest to. He was sharp of wit and intelligence. I don't want to sound partial; I grew to love them all deeply. But Donder was, I guess, special to me. He would show me the things that made each of the others special too. His admiration for each Reindeer was to be reflected in my writing.

The only Reindeer that ever held the special position of lead Reindeer were Donder and Blitzen. The others were positioned any way they wanted to be. Dasher, who was prone to veer to the right a little too much, might slip into the harness on the left of Dancer —who would compensate for Dasher's slight pull to the right. Or Dasher might stay to the right of the harness if the night route called for a Southwest direction. It was all very complicated, as I found out during my stay with these remarkable Christmas Reindeer. Yet to them it was as simple as 1-2-3.

Santa cupped the muzzle of the third Reindeer and looked up laughing. "Comet, the fastest of my Reindeer. Once while returning home, he outdistanced Halley's Comet. I sometimes let the Reindeer out of the harness during the homecoming run so they can stretch their legs and shake the soreness of the traces from their backs.

"On that particular night, around 1834, I had let them all loose except Donder, who maintained control of the sleigh. Of course, they all began to run free in front of the sleigh, glad to be rid of the harness, and just having a good time frolicking. Comet, who was out in front of the pack, sighted the comet and took off after it. He was either too far ahead to respond to my calls, or he just felt so good that he didn't pay any attention to me. He was heading straight for the comet!

"The sight of stardust from his hooves was amazing. For a moment, I thought there were two comets instead of one! He caught up with the comet and soon began to pull ahead of it. That's how he got his name. Even now, I still have a hard time holding him back. Whoever is in front of Comet had better step lively, or his hooves might get trampled on!"

Next, he pointed out: "Now, this is Vixen, my shy Reindeer." The small, but very stout, Reindeer looked up at me and slowly lowered her antlers. Then she looked at me again. I learned from Santa that Vixen was one of the two female Reindeer, the other being Cupid.

"You might say that Vixen keeps everyone in line when they feel overly frisky. If they want to zigzag for the sake of zigzagging, she is the one who promptly scolds them and strictly orders them back into a straight line. She saved all of us one year as we barely cleared Mt. Everest!" Santa rubbed Vixen just behind the base of her small antlers.

The next fellow in line looked mischievous. "And this one's name is Dancer. I guess, out of all my Reindeer, he will be the one to watch. He's a great joker, he is, and will go to any lengths to see a good joke through. Do you know that he once talked the others into hiding my sleigh when I had gone down a chimney in Amsterdam? When I came up, the sleigh, the Reindeer, the presents, and everything were gone! Now that was a fright!

"At first I thought they had been Reindeer-napped. As I sat and pondered this prospect, I could just make out Vixen's voice far across town, scolding Dancer. An awful time she gave him, too. Dancer likes his jokes, but his sense of direction is remarkable. We have never been lost." Santa assured me that Vixen kept her eyes constantly on Dancer and would see that I was not harassed by his jokes.

Santa reached for the next Reindeer. "This solid black fellow with a white mouth is Prancer, first cousin to Dancer. He joined our team some 1,100 years ago when he convinced me that the proof is in the puller. It was Prancer who pulled us all out when the sleigh had become lodged in a glacier and the rest of the Reindeer had frozen solid to the ice. Prancer was the only one who had free footing, and pull he did. If he hadn't we might still be there, frozen in the ice. Prancer is a serious fellow when business needs to be accomplished; and he's not one to fool around. He's a by-the-book Reindeer who will never let you down." Prancer looked pleased at Santa's words.

As we moved to the last two Reindeer in Santa's team, I instinctively knew that the next one would be Dasher. He *looked* like a Dasher, if a name implies anything. He was built for fast sprints and quick takeoffs. He was muscled up a little more than the other Reindeer—except for Donder, who was by far the strongest.

"You've guessed that this is Dasher. He is the fastest Reindeer on takeoff that I have ever encountered. He is quick to respond to the reins and can turn on a dime. He can run straight up the side of a cliff a mile high—and back down again, in the blink of an eye. The load we carry every Christmas Eve is enormous, and Dasher is the one who gets us started on each takeoff. His powerful legs get the sleigh started, and then the rest of the Reindeer take over. His sudden burst of energy is amazing, especially taking off from a narrow, short rooftop. Couldn't do without Dasher, no sir." I could see that Dasher stood on powerful legs of pride, as a privileged member of Santa's team.

Santa then dropped to one knee and hugged the last and smallest of the Reindeer. She looked up at me with curious eyes, and then drank in Santa's affection. She was a soft creature with delicate fur. I wondered how this small Reindeer could possibly keep up with the others.

He whispered in her ear, "Without you, Christmas would not be possible." The littlest Reindeer wriggled ever so slightly and leaned heavily into Santa's shoulder.

"This is Cupid," Santa said, getting to his feet, but keeping one hand on the small Reindeer's head. "Cupid is the youngest, and she sometimes feels that she doesn't pull her own weight. But she's young, and the young sometimes doubt themselves. After all, she's only 719 years old! She tries to stay next to Dasher most of the time, feeling that he will make up for her lack in a long, hard pull. Yet she can pull the sleigh by herself on a level run and has the endurance of 50 average reindeer," he said proudly.

"Cupid is remarkable for seeing that the rest of the Reindeer are hooked up and hitched securely into their traces. She sees to it that all of them take their flight vitamins before each journey. And she's a great morale booster, praising each Reindeer in flight." She beamed proudly at Santa's words.

Santa whispered to me, "Cupid looks to Dasher as a sort of big brother. Dasher always gets special attention when he steps into his traces beside her."

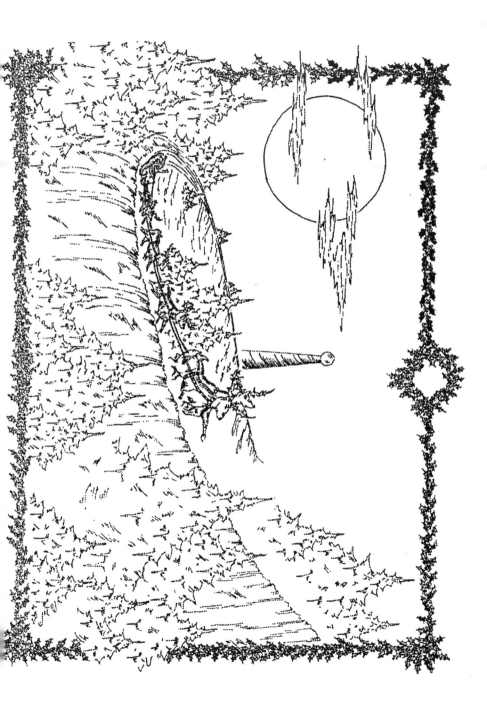

Santa moved toward the sleigh with his arm over my shoulder. He motioned for me to climb aboard.

"Come, Lad, there is much to do, and you must learn how to listen. I can tell that my Reindeer are pleased with you and what you mean to do. There's much to see and accomplish—so we must away!"

With those words, Santa slightly lifted the reins and I felt myself grip the side of the seat beside him. I watched with wonder as the ground and forest below us seemed to grow farther and farther away, and Santa steered the sleigh due north.

In front of us, the magical Christmas Reindeer waltzed on the wind-currents of the night sky.

2

Cupid's Dilemma

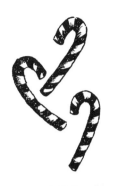

My mind was ablaze with wonder and confusion. I wasn't dreaming! I was actually sitting in a sleigh with Santa Claus, and we were being pulled through the sky by eight flying Reindeer! These were the very eight Reindeer that I was going to write about!

As a child, I always thought I would be awfully cold if I ever got the chance to ride in Santa's sleigh. But it wasn't cold at all. Brisk, maybe, but not the freezing chill I had expected.

Why, not moments before I had been walking in freezing rain, sad and lonely, not caring that it was Christmas Eve. Now I was 10,000 feet in the sky, sitting behind eight magical Reindeer—and beside Santa Claus.

There was no room for doubt. And since I had never really stopped believing in the magic of childhood and Christmas and Santa—I knew it was all real.

Santa's Christmas Eve! And I was a part of it! I wasn't at home in bed waiting for it—I was in the thick of it.

The Reindeer kept a steady rhythm as they swayed to the wind. Each hoof was put down in exactly the right place; each Reindeer was exactly in tune with the others. I watched as sparks of stardust came from each hoof. The stardust trail they and the sleigh left behind them was long as we continued on through the night. Santa, watching my amazement, laughed loud and long.

"Well, Lad, first stop just ahead," pointed out Santa. I saw a small village just before us and to the right. The sleigh began to bank sharply and we lost altitude as we dropped fast into the night sky. I gripped the seat tighter, and my stomach rose sharply too, as I thought we might crash. I felt as though I was trapped inside an elevator in which the cables had broken. We must have been doing better than 500 miles per hour when Santa steered the Reindeer toward a very, very small rooftop.

He pulled back very slowly on the reins. Blitzen, up ahead, began to brake the team and sleigh. I was showered in stardust as the backwind caught up with us. For a moment, I was blinded by the brilliant burst of silvery spray. I saw the rooftop come up at us in superfast motion, like a video camera being put into fast-forward.

I heard Vixen trill sharply with her voice, and all of the Reindeer came to a full-braking power. We gently landed on that very small rooftop. A soft thump, and the touchdown of 32 star-flecked hooves ...and then stillness. Santa looked at me and laughed heartily. I must have looked a sight. Donder told me later that my hair was on end, and I had gripped the side of the sleigh so tightly with my hands that it would need repainting!

"Adjust, Lad, adjust. You'll get used to it. They know what they're doing. Put your trust in them," Santa said with a wave of his arm that included all the Reindeer.

I saw Dancer, the joker, laughing silently out of the corner of his mouth. I would definitely have to keep my eyes on Dancer.

Santa leaned back behind him and pulled out an enormous pack, bulging with presents. Jumping out of the sleigh atop the roof, he slung the pack over his shoulder and, winking at me, said, "Back in a flash. You can start getting acquainted with them now. There'll be more time later, after deliveries. But for now, you can chat and try to get a grip on what you need to write down."

Santa returned to the chimney, and just before disappearing in a swirl of stardust, turned to Dancer. "Behave yourself, or Vixen will ride beside you next year." Laughing, Santa disappeared down the chimney. I looked at Dancer, who was looking hard at Vixen.

"You know, he means it, Dancer," she said. "I would look *forward* to it. Why, it's been almost four hundred years since we teamed together side by side." And she grinned slyly, making Dancer cringe. She might have been shy, but she knew how to keep the other Reindeer on their hooves.

A soft, almost quiet rippling of laughter went through all of the Reindeer—except Blitzen, who was quietly dozing.

"Who's got it? Who's got it?"

I assumed Dasher had said this, as they were looking at him questioningly. Before I forget to put this down, let me try to explain how each Christmas Reindeer can talk, and how I can understand them. Of course, it's magic! You must believe in it. Each Reindeer had a strong accent of his or her own, which I will tell you about later.

Dasher repeated his question. *"Who's got it?* You all know what I'm talking about. Cupid, weren't you chosen this year to do it?"

In front of where I sat in the sleigh, Cupid spoke very quietly, almost nervously. "I've got it, but I really don't think we should. Remember how mad he got last year when we turned the list over to Mrs. Claus?"

Donder, who had quickly unhooked his traces and was sitting in the snow, said, "Sure, he got mad, but he really didn't mean it. He knows we do it for his own good. After all, it's what Mrs. Claus asked us to do. He understands that and doesn't blame us."

Prancer, the serious Reindeer, just shook his head and said, "We don't have time for that. We'd better leave well enough alone."

I couldn't stand it anymore, so I interrupted them. "What are you talking about?" I asked.

Dancer laughed, then quickly looked at Vixen. She just shook her head and said, "You tell him."

"Well," Dancer said, "about 450 years ago, or was it 470? Anyway, Mrs. Claus came to us just as we were about to leave on our Christmas Eve trip. She asked us to keep a list of all the cookies, fruitcakes, eggnog, candy, and whatever else was lying around on tables in the houses we visit—you know, the stuff that Santa eats when he is putting presents under the tree. Didn't you ever leave any milk and cookies or anything for Santa to eat when he came to your house on Christmas Eve?"

"Of course, I did. I always tried to leave chocolate chip cookies and hot cocoa for him. It was always gone in the morning—with a real nice letter from him, thanking me for the snack," I said.

Somehow, I had the feeling that maybe I did something wrong by leaving Santa food to eat on Christmas Eve. The Reindeer, with their uncanny perception, seemed to sense what I was thinking.

"Well, hey," said Comet, "you didn't do anything wrong. Everyone does it. Santa has come to expect it every now and then. Better yet, we even get some of the goodies too. And we also leave thank-you letters to the kids."

"The point is," interrupted Dancer, "Mrs. Claus was becoming quite concerned with all the sweets Santa would eat on Christmas Eve. She asked quite simply if we would keep track of what he eats. So each year we draw straws to see who will list all of the snacks that he consumes. This year, Cupid lost and has to do it."

It seemed to me that Cupid looked absolutely miserable about the task that she had to perform. Then an idea struck me.

"Listen, Cupid," I said. "Would it hurt if I kept the list instead of you? Of course, I can't tell what he is eating down there, but you can tell me, and I'll write it down."

Cupid seemed to brighten somewhat and eagerly nodded her head. Donder, who was scratching his ear, said, "You'll have to write fast. We travel awfully quickly, and he'll be back in a moment. Cupid, you tell him what Santa has wolfed down so far..."

"*Donder,*" said Vixen, horrified. "Santa doesn't *wolf down*—he nibbles."

Dancer started laughing. "*Nibbles?* Vixen, have you seen his belt lately? He's down to the last notch. You don't get in that shape by nibbling! *Wolfing* is the only way to get down to the last notch!"

Donder cleared his throat. "As I was saying, Cupid, you tell the lad what to write and that will more or less let you off the hook. Problem solved. *Agreed?*"

I smiled at Donder. "Agreed."

Down below us, in the house, I could hear soft laughter.

"Does Santa always laugh whenever he goes down a chimney?" I asked no one in particular.

Prancer turned to look at me. "Of course he does, he's Santa Claus."

Dasher grinned. "Lighten up, Prance. It's Lad's first trip out. A lot of this is really new to him. Give him some slack."

I looked at Dasher gratefully as Donder added, "Don't mind Prance. He's all business when deliveries start. He's really a very likable Reindeer. You'll have to get him to take you up to Snowball Hill when we get home. He holds the record for the biggest snowball, right Prancer?"

"Why, yes," smiled Prancer. "I'll be glad to escort him to Snowball Hill if he would like to go."

"Prancer," I said, "I would be honored to go there with you." I felt a small hoof on my arm and turned to see Cupid.

"Get ready to write. Santa's found the goodies. Oh, mercy, let's see: four mint cookies, two glasses of milk, a ham on rye, hold the mayo, and a small piece of fruitcake. That's all."

Cupid smiled up at me as I feverishly wrote down the list of what Santa had eaten.

"My goodness," I said. "Is this only our first stop of the night?" I really didn't think Santa would eat like that at every stop. I thought maybe he had missed his supper before they took off.

"That's nothing," said Dancer, laughing. "Wait till

we hit the Bering Sea. That's the last leg of our journey. You take a look at that snack list then!"

"Wolfing..." Donder giggled.

"Dancer, Donder, show some respect," scolded Vixen. "Santa enjoys his snacks."

Up front, still sitting in the snow, Donder said, "You bet he does. Everyone thinks the sleigh is fairly light when we head for home. No way! As the presents go out, the snacks come in, and the sleigh takes on quite a bit of weight. We broke a runner three years ago when we landed on that little girl's home in French Guiana. She writes a nice letter. She also left us some tasty snacks."

Comet smiled and said, "It's nothing we can't handle, though. Santa has a way of throwing off most of that weight before we make it home. I don't know how he does it. Magic, maybe. But he's about the same size when we get home as he was when we left. No problem."

A rustling at the chimney interrupted us, and Santa was again in the sleigh with a broad smile on his face.

"Getting to know each other, Lad?" he asked.

"They are amazing Reindeer," I said, laughing.

"That they are, Lad. That they are." With a careful, thoughtful glance at Cupid, Santa touched the reins that brought Blitzen out of his nap. Once again we were on our way to the next rooftop.

3

A High-Climb Run and Grandfather Blitzen

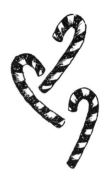

We traveled fast and far that magical night, and I don't think there was ever a dull moment. I listened to Vixen scold Dancer... watched as Blitzen took a hundred naps... witnessed an amazing sprint race between Comet and Dasher across two states in the Southwestern part of America—while Santa worked overtime at a condominium complex.

I listened in awe as Prancer told me in detail the art of making the biggest snowballs back home. I later mastered this accomplishment with excellent tutoring from Prancer.

Cupid continued to give me the list of snacks and goodies that Santa ate. The list was growing steadily longer. I began to wonder if I would have enough paper to keep up with it all. Cupid assured me (reading my thoughts again) that there was an ample amount of paper and pens in the sleigh glove compartment in front of me.

There was a series of dials and glowing buttons across the front of the "dash" of the sleigh. They constantly blinked off and on, and from time to time emitted a soft hum. When we stopped in Winnipeg, Donder explained to me that this was the radar detection equipment that Santa had had installed about 50 years earlier. It would alert him and his Reindeer to UFOs, jumbo-jets, satellites, and ice clouds—not to mention strong wind-currents that would sometimes push them off course a couple of miles or more.

Dancer, I found out, had been a little put out by all this scientific equipment. He had argued that his sense of direction was fail-safe. After several years of experimenting, Santa had agreed that no piece of equipment could replace Dancer's built-in instincts and radar. Santa had retained the equipment in case Dancer should fall ill with the flu some year and not be able to make the trip.

Dancer had protested. The other Reindeer had jumped on him in private, away from Santa's ears. They told Dancer to be quiet about the equipment. These were Santa's toys. Dancer had reluctantly succumbed to modern technology.

Actually, Santa himself is just a big kid, and, while a teddy bear or a toy drum would make him happy, I always noticed a glow of special satisfaction when he was playing with his radar detector. He was just like any grown man playing with toy trains. Yet Dancer continued to resent those pieces of glow-in-the-dark gadgets, seeing them as an insult to his never-get-lost instincts.

As we buzzed our way across South America, I wrote quickly. Trying to keep up with Reindeer dialogue, and taking down Cupid's list of snacks, was beginning to take its toll on me—a mere mortal who had been handed a miracle so many hours ago in the freezing rain.

I must mention that wherever we went, it was snowing. There was always a soft, thick bed of snow for the sleigh to land on. Even in the South Pacific atolls, where we were so close to the equator and the temperature must have been 100 degrees, it still felt brisk, like a frost that covered the morning grass.

Prancer, the serious-minded Reindeer, explained that no matter where they went, they carried the spirit of Christmas magic with them. Each house, no matter how humble, would be touched with Christmas snow. This was because Reindeer could not pull very long when the temperature was above 80 degrees. So an automatic thermostat control had been installed in the sleigh some 900 years earlier, to make it possible for Santa and his magical team of Reindeer to carry Christmas snow directly from the North Pole.

I thought, how wonderful that each home can be blessed with the spirit of Christmas magic! These Reindeer and Santa could see that every child got a taste of it, even if just for a moment once a year.

Yet I quickly learned that not only small children were included in this Christmas magic, but older ones—and grownups as well.

"You aren't grownups," explained Vixen thoughtfully. "Just bigger children!"

I felt nearly bursting with happiness. She was right! "Something to think about, huh?" said Vixen with a sparkle in her eyes.

As we soared across the night sky and headed due northeast, toward England, we picked up speed. Everyone was laughing loudly now, even Santa.

Blitzen sprang to life in time to see the clear, moonlit sea beneath us, and the waves making crescent sparkles as the moonbeams hit them. It was breathtaking... And the wind—oh, the wind! It rushed by us, roaring the silent roar of a thousand eddies. Although

I could feel it, it wasn't pushing against us as I had expected. It was just a calm breeze. But the speed at which we were traveling left me breathless.

As if Donder read my thoughts, he yelled back to Dasher, "What about it, Dash, can you give us some more speed?"

As if a challenge had been accepted, Dasher strained and I could see the muscled knots stand out on his powerful legs. With a sudden spurt forward, stronger than I would have thought possible, the sleigh gained even more momentum. Comet, sensing the chase, strained for all he was worth, and still more speed was gained. We flew over the waves in a blur, the stardust blistering out behind us like fiery flames.

Santa, laughing so hard I thought he would burst, leaned toward me and said, "Watch ol' Blitzen. They think they've finally got him. They think that because of his age he won't be able to keep up with Dasher and Comet."

I watched Blitzen closely, hoping with all my might that the old fellow could keep up with the maddening speed with which Dasher and Comet pulled. As if in answer to my thoughts, the aged Christmas Reindeer slowly turned his massive antlers and head slightly toward me. Out of the corner of his eye, he winked at me, and I saw an ever-so-slight grin touch the corners of his mouth. Then, looking forward again, he lowered his majestic antlers slightly. I felt the sleigh give a sudden jerk forward, and the race was on! Of course, there was nothing to race against but each other, and Blitzen was going to give those two rascally young Reindeer a run for their candy canes.

"*Yahooo!*" screamed Dasher. "*He's awake now! Show*

us how it's done, Grandfather! Comet and I will soon catch you!"

The stardust trail lengthened for miles as the old Reindeer poured it on. Donder was screaming for more when Blitzen banked hard to the left and began to climb. Upward we climbed with the same accelerating speed. The stars seemed to welcome us as we hit the outer atmosphere. Still, Blitzen showed no signs of slowing down. He had been challenged, and even Santa's frantic tugging on the reins failed to slow him down. In disgust, Santa dropped the reins and leaned back, smiling at me.

"When he gets like this, I can only let him run his own course," said Santa. "My bet is that he will soon have Comet and Dasher begging for mercy. Only then will he back off and let Dancer get us back on course. Still, it's great fun, isn't it?" Having said that, Santa began to cheer Blitzen on with shouts of encouragement: *"Away, Blitzen, away!"*

I didn't know if I could stand this kind of fun much longer. The round horizon of earth was visible now, and I had some serious doubts about ever returning there. Still, Blitzen pushed forward, climbing ever higher—until I thought I might reach out and grab a star. Comet began to show small signs of tiring. Dasher, who was excellent in the short, hard sprints, was covered in perspiration, his sides heaving. He was frantically trying to keep up with the maddening pace that Blitzen had set for them. Frightened, I looked at Santa, who was taking his break, as he called it, to down a carton of eggnog he had somehow slipped past the ever-watchful Cupid.

"He'll make them both say 'uncle' before he quits," said Santa, grinning. "Then, he'll still climb a few more miles to give them something to think about. Happens every year. Those two, Comet and Dasher, always play this game with Blitzen on Christmas Eve. And they know he looks forward to it, although he would never admit it.

"I think it's a wonderful kind of love they show ol' Blitzen. A love you will better understand the more time you spend with them. If you haven't noticed, Lad, those two can't see a thing in front of them. They have relied entirely on Blitzen. Blitzen knows that and loves them for it. Blitzen may nap on a rooftop now and again, but he knows that when the chips are down, those two will stand behind him, no matter what."

At that very instant, I heard the two Reindeer scream, "*Uncle!*"

We climbed a few more miles at the same speed, then suddenly Blitzen banked hard to the right and began a long descent. Blitzen turned toward Dancer and muttered something. I realized that Blitzen had given Dancer his cue to chart our path and bring the team back on the correct course.

Dancer began a series of high-winded sniffings, shaking his big antlers from right to left in his efforts to turn the team once again toward England. I noticed a shift in the sleigh. The Reindeer, following Dancer's lead, pulled and tugged once again. As we entered the lower atmosphere, I could make out England on our right. Santa, seeing land, took the reins and slowly turned the sleigh even more, pulling back ever so slightly to give the Reindeer a rest before entering London.

We circled Big Ben, just for the fun of it, then set down in Liverpool. The sleigh came to a rest softly on the first row of buildings that Santa was to visit. Santa grabbed his pack and hopped out.

"I'll be gone a while, so take a breather and get your hooves back on the ground." He turned toward a very skinny chimney, paused, and looked back. "For your information, Cupid, the boy who lives here with his younger sister always leaves me a nice, juicy, sweet, thick, *large* slice of fruitcake. Their names are Joe and Linda, and they make the cake themselves. Should be about 2,600 calories—and I'm going to enjoy every bite of it!"

I quickly wrote down that Reindeer *do* turn red from embarrassment, as I observed from Cupid's reaction.

Santa quickly patted her head, then disappeared down the chimney, laughing.

"I really didn't think he knew," said Cupid, looking at me.

"Of course he does, he's Santa Claus," broke in Prancer.

Donder had unhooked himself and was lying spread-eagle in the snow, panting. "By the great Borealis, Grandfather, that was fantastic!"

Blitzen, who was starting to doze, opened one eye at Donder and whispered, *"Ahyup."*

"Comet, you're not saying much. Want me to rub your tired, sore back for you?" asked Vixen. She said this with a little too much sarcasm, judging by the look on Comet's face.

Vixen continued, "Oh, Dasher, I hope your hooves don't hurt too much."

"Try not to trouble yourself so much about my hooves, thank you. I was just about to get my second wind," Dasher answered, sounding hurt.

"Right on, you guys. That must be why you two almost blew my antlers off when I heard that frantic scream of *'Uncle!'*" Dancer said, sitting down in his traces in the snow, his sides heaving with laughter.

I was wishing I had my tape recorder. I couldn't write fast enough to get down all of their dialogue. Donder stood up and shook the sweat off his sides.

"Who's afraid of the big, bad Blitzen, right, Comet?"

"Oh, go... go stuff your stocking," said Comet, trying to ignore Donder's remark.

Although the banter went back and forth from Reindeer to Reindeer, and Blitzen was quietly dozing through all of their joking, I could feel their real affection for the old Reindeer. Blitzen had once again proved that he was still King of the Sky. For all of their joking and good-natured insults, I could see and feel from each of them that the first and oldest Reindeer was still their hero. They would have no other lead them through the magical skies of Christmas Eve.

Cupid had slipped her traces and moved quietly up front where she gently adjusted the old king's ear traces so that they wouldn't hang down over his ears. She lovingly tucked his shoulder harness snugly down around his flanks. Even now, Blitzen showed no sign of fatigue or the heavy breathing that Comet and Dasher were experiencing.

Cupid leaned slightly upward and gently kissed the old Reindeer on his gray, muzzled cheek, and gave him an equally gentle hug around his massive shoulders. Grandfather Blitzen murmured in his sleep and smiled. Cupid silently tiptoed back to her own place in the harness. The others nodded their approval and talked more quietly, so as not to disturb his nap.

Wiping her eyes quickly, Cupid looked at me and whispered, "And that's why he is Grandfather Blitzen. That's why we all love him so. He is the oldest and first chosen, and no matter how old he becomes, if he shows any sign that pulling or leading his team would be even a slight hardship, there's not one of us who wouldn't carry him through the night skies on our mission.

"Try to understand, he is the Grandfather to us. We take our problems to him when we are bothered or troubled. He freshens our spirits and inspires us with his kindness and gentleness. He would never let us down—and certainly would never disappoint the children. He would step aside before he would let that happen. I think that's why every Christmas Eve run, Comet and Dasher try to renew his sense of worth with a good high-climb run."

Cupid smiled and wiped her eyes again. "It will take him several days to rest from this one, though. And even tonight…" Cupid quickly bit her quivering lower lip. "I could feel the ever-so-slight extra pull that Donder was giving him. What I'm trying to say is, had Grandfather aimed for the moon tonight, there's not one among us who wouldn't have seen to it that he succeeded in his pull toward the heavens. He would have collapsed rather than fallen. Comet and Dasher knew when to say 'Uncle,' although tonight he gave them more than they bargained for. He definitely gave them a run for their candy canes! That was the best high-climb run I have experienced in three-score and fifteen years."

Cupid smiled gently. "Tonight, he was the Blitzen of Christmas Eves we remember so well of a thousand years past. Santa knew it too, and I think Grandfather will find an extra goodie in his stocking tomorrow morning when he wakes. And not just from Santa, but from all of us. He'll make light of it, of course, and put it off as nothing. But he'll be pleased. Oh, yes, he'll be ever so pleased."

I felt tears welling up inside me. Now I had even more respect and admiration for Blitzen, the first-chosen Christmas Reindeer.

The other Reindeer stood silently, as Cupid whispered to me. When she had finished, they all bowed their heads in respect. Never had I felt such closeness and love.

Silently, I gave thanks that I had been allowed to share in this Christmas magic.

4

A Christmas Gift for Grandfather Blitzen

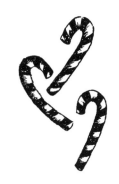

When Santa returned, he was bearing gifts for the Reindeer—a sack of cookies and other goodies he had picked up during his deliveries. As Santa distributed to each Reindeer what he thought each one would like, I saw him fondly stroke Blitzen's chest and offer him a piece of fruitcake. Nodding his thank-you, Blitzen began to eat.

Santa moved back to the sleigh and sat down beside me. Leaning forward, he interrupted Cupid's munching of an extremely large Christmas cookie and said, "I was wrong about that piece of fruitcake, Cupid. They left me *three* pieces."

Santa turned to me and asked, "Did you get that down, Lad?" Nodding to indicate that I had, but not revealing that Cupid had informed me earlier of the extra piece of fruitcake, I pretended to write this down.

Santa looked thoughtfully at his notes, and, I think, surprised everyone by saying, "Tonight, instead of traveling due east through Scotland and Italy, we will turn south toward Africa. Then we'll fly across the Indian Ocean, go through India, and circle back through Russia. Dancer, would you please compute our course. I want us to be on our way."

Dancer began a sort of vague humming sound that I later discovered was his way of allowing no distractions to interfere with his lightning-fast course changes. Dancer automatically knew what route Santa wanted to take when he changed his mind.

Within a minute, Dancer turned to Santa and nodded that he was ready. He had the course imprinted in his mind. With a yell that brought all the Reindeer to their feet, and their ears turned forward, Santa tugged at the reins: *"Away, Blitzen... away!"*

We were off once again. We covered Spain with lightning speed; the presents and toys were now safely beneath the Christmas trees in each home.

There wasn't a lot of talking among the Reindeer, except for an occasional, "Don't crowd me" or "Get off my hoof."

We traveled fast, and I somehow knew we had lost a little time with our high-climbing flight over the Atlantic Ocean. The Reindeer had sensed this also, and were all business now as we soared over the Mediterranean Sea, toward the coast of Africa.

Down through Algeria, Libya, Egypt—crisscrossing to catch Mali, Sudan, and Nigeria. We flew south toward Tanzania, Angola, and Mozambique, and then into South Africa. We took a much-needed break in Johannesburg. We saw Santa disappear into the doorway of a small home.

The moment he was out of view, Cupid began her recitation of goodies he had consumed, exclaiming, "He'd better slow down. He's not going to leave us much if he doesn't slow down."

I frantically recorded what was disappearing below. I looked at Cupid in amazement as she quipped, "Two bowls of vegetable soup."

I stammered, "Is that what the children left for him?"

"Oh, no," said Cupid. "He's already finished the sandwich and milk that were left out for him. He's in the kitchen now. Oh, oh... make that *three* bowls of vegetable soup."

Cupid grinned. "That's our Santa!"

From the front of the sleigh, I could hear Vixen telling Dancer that "Yes, the lost time has been made up," and "No, *we aren't going to do it!*"

Dancer had to be up to one of his tricks, I thought. I leaned forward to catch the conversation that even Donder and Comet had now joined. I thought Dancer looked especially sly with a piece of straw hanging from the corner of his muzzle—he was using it for a toothpick.

Donder looked from Comet to Vixen and grumbled, "Aw, what's the harm? We won't be gone long. Anyway, he's got all the presents he needs for the short time it would take us."

Vixen began to waver. After all, wasn't Donder the second-lead Reindeer? He always made rational decisions. Vixen turned to Dasher and Cupid and asked, "What do you think?"

Dasher grinned and Cupid giggled.

"Settled, then!" said Dancer. "Let's go."

As Dasher began to dig in, I stood up and yelled, "*Wait a minute, you guys!* What's going on? You can't just take off and leave Santa!"

Too late! We were already crossing the Natal Basin and moving fast. The speed at which we took off made me sit down abruptly and desperately grip the sides of the sleigh. The water flew by under us and we skirted islands that looked like mere dots below.

"*Donder—what's happening!!?*" I screamed. I didn't dare move very much as the sleigh was beginning to turn and rock. Without the added weight of Santa and all those snacks, the Reindeer were almost weightless.

I realized that the sleigh was picking up speed. We suddenly hit strong wind turbulence, and the sleigh tipped crazily on its side, and then righted itself.

"*Not to worry, Lad!*" yelled Donder over his shoulder. "We're going to plunge through the Tropic of Capricorn and catch a star to put in Blitzen's stocking. He has only one left, and it's starting to fade. We thought we'd get him another one—should last him several hundred years."

I would find out later that stars were very important to Christmas Reindeer. They mostly favored the red stars, but a blue star was a prize—they were the hardest to find.

Of course I wouldn't worry! After all, we had just left Santa Claus 2,000 miles behind us. We were riding wind-currents at 10,000 feet, and the sleigh was starting to rock and roll without the added weight of Santa. I remembered that I had also joined in eating the snacks that Santa had brought back when we were in Liverpool.

Throughout the twisting and turning, I could see that Blitzen was still napping. Donder, and Comet (having hooked into Blitzen's traces), were gently carrying him through the wind-currents.

I felt utterly helpless! This was another one of Dancer's escapades! Dancer had talked them all into it.

Had Santa left me in charge while he was gone? I didn't think so. I was just an innocent bystander caught up in the pranks of eight Christmas Reindeer. Excuse me—*seven* Reindeer. Blitzen was asleep. I wondered what he would have thought about this if he had awakened.

Cupid turned to me. "He won't wake up. Donder has pushed some cumulus clouds under him as we're flying. He'll sleep as though he were home for awhile —at least long enough for us to get what we came for."

I heard Comet yell, "Straight ahead—to the right, six degrees! A big one, and moving fast!!"

Prancer, who had joined in because he really had no choice, moved his head to the outside for a quick look.

"Quickly, Donder," yelled Prancer. "It's a *blue* one. Dive! Dive!"

I felt the sleigh give way from under me as Donder began to dive like a falcon, followed by the other Reindeer. I could see the star now! The Reindeer had taught me a thing or two about eyesight. I was curled around the right sleigh runner, holding on tightly. I had lost my grip when Donder had plunged through the Tropic of Capricorn with the speed of a bullet. We were gaining on the star, a bright blue one that was leaving a sparkling trail miles in length...

In the midst of this frantic pursuit, Dasher yelled for me to look under the seat of the sleigh. There I would find a crimson red star-bag made of heavy material.

"Sure," I thought. "We're just going 12,000 miles per hour. I'm hanging on for dear life to the right sleigh runner. The seat of the sleigh is only five feet above me. Why don't I just skip up there and get the bag? While I'm at it, why don't I just let go and fall about four miles and take a nice, cold bath in the Indian Ocean?"

Cupid reached back with her right hoof. Never missing a step in their all-out pursuit of the star, she righted the sleigh so I could scramble back in. Once back in the safety of the seat, I reached for the bag, and my fingers soon clutched at its drawstrings. I pulled it out from under the seat and held onto it.

Dasher saw that I had it and yelled, "When Donder sweeps under the star, open the drawstrings and pull the bag up behind it! Close the bag quickly so it doesn't get away! Be careful not to touch it, if you can help it!"

I was just about ready to go through with this, having gotten my courage up, when Dasher had said, "Don't touch it." I soon saw why.

The closer we got to the star, the more the immediate surroundings of the sleigh—and we ourselves—began to glow with a brilliant blue. I could just barely make out the shapes of the Reindeer through the shiny, blue haze.

"*If you touch it,*" Dasher screamed through the glimmer, "*you'll become weightless and won't be able to hold yourself in the sleigh.*"

"*Nowwwww!*" screamed Donder. There was no time to think about it. I leaned out of the sleigh with the bag open and watched, terrified, as the brilliant star moved closer and closer. I hooked my left leg around the left side of the sleigh and hung suspended in space. Donder did a tricky, sweeping dive, and I had the star! It was wiggling frantically in the sack. I quickly drew in the drawstrings and the sky once again returned to its normal color of dark blue.

I felt the wind rushing by as Donder did an about-face turn in the sky. The extra push from all the Reindeer—except Blitzen, who was still napping—righted the sleigh. We were once again headed back the way we had come, toward South Africa.

I tied the bag holding the precious blue star, held it secure, and looked up at the Reindeer. They were all covered with a shiny, blue haze. And I was too. The sleigh looked as though it had been given a bath in blue glitter.

In spite of the way we looked, and the scolding Santa would surely give us—I grinned from ear to ear and laughed loudly. All the Reindeer turned in their traces to see what was going on.

"We did it!" I screamed. "We did it!" This set all of them to laughing so hard that the sleigh began to weave again. Their laughing subsided somewhat. And Prancer, who had so eagerly joined in the pursuit, said, "Now, my fine Christmas Reindeer, how do we explain blue stardust all over us and Santa's sleigh?"

That's when we all heard the low growl of Grandfather Blitzen. No one knew how long he had been awake. Cupid gave a groan. "We've had it now!"

"I thought he was asleep," hissed Comet, looking hard at Donder.

Donder kept his eyes straight ahead, not daring to look at Blitzen, and whispered, "I thought he was, too."

I felt the sleigh turn to the right, and I knew Grandfather Blitzen was pulling us now.

I heard Blitzen say through gritted teeth, "A fine thing to show our guest. Behaving like Christmas imps. Now you've gotten us covered with stardust. Blue, too, it seems."

With this, Blitzen gave a thoughtful grumble. "Follow my lead, Donder, you young scamp. The rest of you keep step, and I'll rid us of this worrisome stardust."

The sleigh picked up speed, and Blitzen started

leading the Reindeer through a series of turns that had me holding on for dear life. We must have looked like a drill bit at full speed, as we turned with as much speed corkscrewing as we had going forward.

The sky lit up with blue haze as the stardust began to fling itself off the Reindeer and the sleigh. I felt as though I were being turned inside out. Just as fast as Blitzen had started the turning, he began to slow the team down. Needless to say, when Blitzen had straightened us up on the right course, all except Blitzen himself had lost their equilibrium. Their sense of balance was gone! Had it not been for Blitzen, who seemed unaffected by the wild spinning, we might have ended up anywhere.

Donder was turned sideways in the traces, facing Vixen. Comet was upside down and still running, but backwards. Dancer and Prancer were touching tails and running away from each other. Vixen was tangled in her traces and simply being pulled along. Dasher and Cupid just hung together upside down, their legs making feeble attempts at running very slowly.

I had both legs draped over the back of the sleigh and was wondering why my head was pushing against the floorboard.

I imagine we were not a pretty sight as Blitzen pulled the entire weight of the sleigh and the Reindeer with effortless ease.

As they all began to regain their balance, and I did too, they started to straighten out their traces and ease back into formation. Each Reindeer then picked up the step that Blitzen had set for them to follow. I uprighted myself and tried to clear my head. I heard Donder make a sound like a cartoon character, shaking his head from side to side. Then we heard Grand father Blitzen laughing a low, growling laugh, as though he was really enjoying the moment.

"Dancer," Blitzen said, "this is your doing, if I know you." Dancer hung his head.

"Well, you had better get us back on course. I imagine Santa's wondering what has happened to us. As for the rest of you, I would be thinking of a good explanation as to why you left him sitting on a rooftop and took off. Personally, I'm going back to sleep and leaving you to your own resources!"

With that said, Blitzen reached over and hooked his traces into Donder's, and gently lowered his head to nap again.

I must say that it was a sorry-looking bunch that landed on that rooftop. Seeing Santa sitting on the roof's edge stroking his beard made them all hang their heads—even me. I was still clutching the star-bag, with the blue haze still on my hands.

Feeling like criminals caught in the act, we landed. As Santa sat down beside me, he gave the star-bag a thoughtful glance. Taking the reins once again, he tugged them gently and we lifted off toward India and the path we had strayed from.

Blitzen had awakened long enough to look at Santa and nod his head. The word was passed back down the line that, once again, Grandfather Blitzen had covered for all of them. Each Reindeer knew that Blitzen, in his own way of speaking with Santa, had assured him that everything was all right—that they had acted like the youngsters they were, but that now all was forgiven.

With a look of relief on each Reindeer's face, they again picked up their hooves and stepped lively, their hearts once again filled with gladness.

We sped on into the night sky.

5

Children of the Reindeer and Thoughts of Home

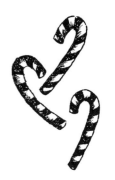

India was a breeze, if I, as a first-trip traveler may say so. It seemed that everything went smoothly. Onward, then, into China, as we followed the Great Wall of China for miles. I found out later that Donder had requested this of Santa so that I might see sights I'd never glimpsed before.

Because I had never seen things that were so common to all of the Christmas Reindeer, it was as though *they, too,* were seeing them for the first time all over again! They all took great pleasure in calling to my attention anything I had not seen before. The writing pads and pens that Santa had placed in the sleigh for me were soon used up.

We stopped in Japan, in a little village called Otaru in the northern part of the country. Santa replenished my supply of writing paper and pens, and we continued on our way. We flew back across the Sea of Japan, into Korea.

I did notice that whenever we entered a country that was divided by war or political movements, there was still no neglecting those children. Each house, hut, shack, or tenement was visited with Christmas in mind. Each dwelling was sprinkled with Christmas snow. Santa entered and left everything that had been asked for on his list that year.

I learned also that Santa might leave a note to each child reminding him or her to be good: not to pull the cat's tail, and to mind their parents, love their neighbors, and improve just a little bit every day.

Each Reindeer perked up as we neared a house that held a special memory. "This is where Tommy lives," Donder said. And Dasher added, "I see that Susan left her bicycle outside again." The Reindeer busied themselves writing thank-you notes, or even letters, to the thoughtful children who left special treats for them outside their houses. They also left a special sign that these treats were appreciated: they left the ground sparkled with the stardust that had dropped from their fur as they ate.

I especially remember our flight into Tennessee in the United States. I could feel the excitement in each Reindeer as we neared one home that was far from the main town—a small house set far back in the forest. Blitzen, who had not said very much during the trip (he was a Reindeer of few words, but when he spoke, the others listened), cleared his throat and spoke with the sound of bells in his voice.

"They have not forgotten us... bless them," he said.

We landed, not on the rooftop, but by the side of a small frame house. There were mounds of cookies and plenty of sweet milk set outside just for the Reindeer. As the others busied themselves eating, it was Grandfather Blitzen who took paper and pen in hoof and wrote the letter to the little girls who lived there, Laura and Diana. He took quite some time composing his letter, and he paused thoughtfully now and again before continuing his writing.

When he was finished, he placed the letter that had been signed "All of us" on the plate, now empty of cookies. He set the present beside it himself. Then he ate the cookies that Donder had saved for him, while Cupid adjusted his ear traces, which had fallen over his face.

I had stepped out of the sleigh for a moment to stretch my legs. I was chatting with Donder, who had finished his cookies. I inquired about the two little girls who lived here, and the food that had been left out for the Reindeer.

"They have never forgotten, these two dear ones. For six years, we have always found their offering of food for us," Donder said, smiling. "This house may not be blessed with wealth, but it is blessed with faith in *the Christmas belief that we live*, and that each Christmas Eve we journey around the world to bring the children toys.

"At other stops along the way there will be food left for us by other children, but this house is a little different. This family has gone through many hard times. But their belief in us is unshakable. We feel their belief in Christmas magic, even miles from their house. We found their first letter six years ago—almost missed it!

"Blitzen spotted it as we stood on the rooftop. He was the one to read it. When he handed me the letter to read to the others, he turned quickly away. I was sure he was crying, but he wouldn't let anyone see him. Grandfather had been overwhelmed by the love of these two children who had asked us for nothing for themselves, but only for others.

"Blitzen wrote the reply himself, as he has done every Christmas Eve since. He has always left something very special for these two girls. Despite the poverty that surrounds their lives, Grandfather sees to it that they will have something to open on Christmas morning.

Donder wiped his eyes and said, "Grandfather looks forward to this stop every year. He always shakes a little more stardust off his antlers than the others do, so that these two children's eyes will open wide with wonder as they peer out their window to see if we've been here.

"So far, the girls have not disappointed him. And although they are older children now, we always find the food and letters waiting for us. It's that kind of Christmas magic that makes the trips and our jobs worthwhile. For Grandfather, it fills his heart with pride and humility. There are many who don't believe, but we keep trying."

I thought about my own childhood after Donder had finished his story. I had also left food outside for the Reindeer, and had received their thank-you letters. Those letters also had been signed "All of us." I wondered if they had felt my belief in Christmas magic as I had placed the cookies or cake outside for them.

I quickly looked at Blitzen and found that he had turned and was staring straight into my eyes.

"Aye, we felt it, Lad, and that is why you are here." Blitzen smiled and turned back to his cookies. I quickly wiped my eyes and got back into the sleigh.

Cupid turned to me and said, "That's OK. We all feel like that from time to time. There's nothing wrong with it. Think how *hard* we would be if we didn't have such feelings."

As we flew through Korea and then up the coast of Russia on the outskirts of Siberia, there was a quick-

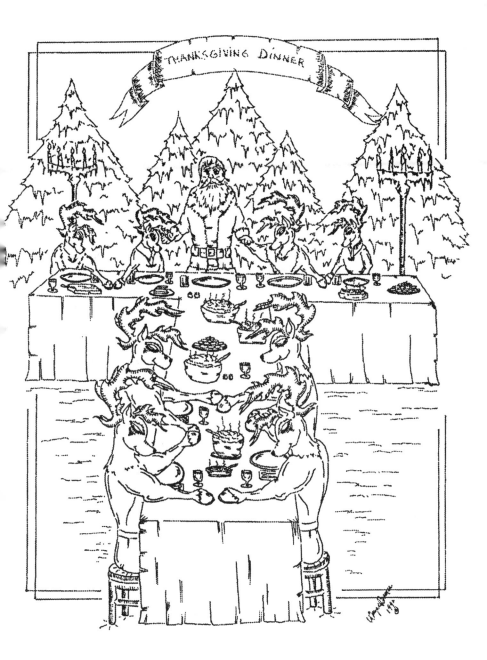

ening pace among all the Reindeer. We were on the last leg of the magical journey. We followed the Arctic Circle, and that's when the carols started. Softly at first, from up front, I believe the first notes came from Donder. I could just hear the chorus of "Jingle Bells."

Comet, then Vixen, started to sing along with Donder. Santa began to tap his big, black boot along with the melody. Before you could say "Christmas tree," we were all singing "Jingle Bells" at the top of our lungs!

Even Blitzen was singing—though, bless his old heart, he couldn't carry a tune in a water bucket. No one cared. It was Christmas Eve! It was snowing, and the air was brisk. It made you shiver 'way down deep, not from the cold, but because of what night this was.

"'Tis the season to be jolly." Each Reindeer was swaying with the melody, and all of their antlers were throwing off thousands of shiny sparkles. We dipped and dived through the night sky. I know we put any roller-coaster to shame. We skimmed the treetops and scattered snow from deep drifts.

We were high in the sky, then low to the ground. All was right with the world on this night, and each Reindeer felt it. Our hearts were lifted as we soared on the wind. We set down just outside of Omsk, where Santa explained to me that he could make his deliveries faster on foot, as the houses were set so close together.

I watched him disappear into the snow, and then bent to my task of trying to organize all of my writings and notes. So far, they had accumulated into a heap in the bottom of the sleigh. As I rifled through the papers I had written, I heard Vixen say, "Don't worry yourself with all of that just now. There'll be plenty of time for that once we reach the Pole."

Children of the Reindeer and Thoughts of Home

Had I heard right? Was I to return with them to the North Pole? The thought had crossed my mind quite a few times since our journey began, but I had not dared to hope for it.

Cupid, who was the closest to me, turned and said firmly, "Of course, you're going home with us. You surely didn't think you could cover everything about us in a single night, did you? You still have to cover our life histories. You know, where we came from, how Santa chose us for his team, our personalities and preferences... all the things I guess a writer must put down when writing about someone."

I was going home! I began to reel with joy. HOME! These magical Christmas Reindeer were going to take me home. I was to see Santa's castle, the elves, the toy factory, Mrs. Claus...

"Throw some more snow on him, quick," yelled Dasher. "He looks like he's going to faint!"

In my joy, I reeled to and fro, almost falling from the sleigh. A soft, cold mush of Siberian-cold snow hit me in the face. That brought me back to consciousness.

"Bullseye!" yelled Dancer.

How did I know that, out of all these Reindeer, Dancer would be the one to hit me with a snowball? I laughed, not caring whether he had buried me in the snow. I was going home!

Comet had slipped his traces, a trick they used quite effectively when they had to. He was thumping me on the back. I looked up and all the Reindeer had gathered around me, smiling and chuckling. Grandfather Blitzen was standing there looking at me and smiling.

"You're the first, you know," said Prancer, "the

first mortal ever to really experience all of this. You will see things unimaginable even in your wildest dreams. But you must be precise in what you report, totally accurate in your writing."

We stood there in the frozen wasteland of Russia, and I felt as though *I had finally been accepted.*

"We really weren't sure, you know, until we saw you in action, leaning out of the sleigh over the Tropic of Capricorn. You chanced everything, just because we told you to do it," said Donder.

Getting that star for Blitzen! The star had been the test they had given me, and I had passed with flying colors. Blue, to be specific. Star blue.

"When do we get there?" I asked loudly. I realized I was shouting and lowered my voice. At least, I *tried* to lower my voice.

Comet was still thumping me on the back, saying, "Calm down, Lad. You'll choke on your own happiness."

Donder hopped up into the sleigh beside me and grinned, saying, "There's Switzerland. Oh, you'll love the Alps. Then Finland, Sweden, Norway... We still have a lot of ground and sky to cover yet. Be patient, we'll get there."

"I pointed to where I thought north was. "Is that the way home?" I asked.

Blitzen answered me in his thick, Scottish accent. "Aye, Lad, a little more to the left." I felt somewhat calmer as I listened to Blitzen. "Follow the star, Lad. The big one that shines so brightly. See it? Good. Now, just under that star is home. There's not one among us who could not find that star and home."

"Is the castle where you live really made of gold and silver?" I eagerly questioned them. My mind was

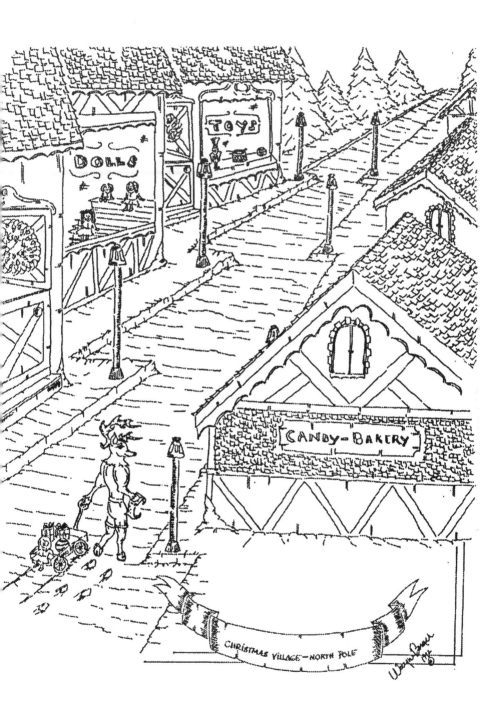

beginning to reel as the questions began to crowd against each other, each wanting to be answered first.

"'Tis a stone castle, not gold or silver, but magic stone, brought from the Middle East, from near the town of Bethlehem. You know of it?" asked Blitzen.

I knew! I knew!

"'Twas Donder and I that carried the magic stone to build the good Santa Claus' castle. The magic was alive in those stones, and still is. 'Twas magic at work as the stones were laid. Magic and love. We can feel it from here, Lad. All of us. It forever draws us to it. No matter where we are, home is just under the Great Star."

I truly felt the magic then, and they all knew it. It was what they had been waiting for. I put my arms around Donder and Comet and hugged them close. The other Christmas Reindeer gathered close around me. I was a part of the magic now. I was going home!

6

An Emergency of Highest Priority

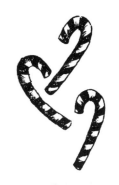

Suddenly a dark form burst through the snow toward us. It was Santa, and he was out of breath. "*Quick*, for Christmas' sake, quick! We have a condition 3! The Alps in East Austria, the Gross Glockner Peak!"

Santa threw his pack of toys into the back of the sleigh and hopped in as he was yelling. The Reindeer immediately hitched up their traces. Cupid scurried from one Reindeer to the next, tightening here and there, paying special attention to Donder and Blitzen. She hooked some sort of special equipment into their side traces—something she had gotten quickly from the back of the sleigh.

"*Hurry, Lassie,*" shouted Santa. "*Hurry!* We haven't much time!"

Cupid was working frantically now with Blitzen's traces and side harness. Donder moved in closer to Blitzen and helped to brace the heavy ropes that Cupid had draped from his massive shoulders.

The rest of the team, at a signal from Comet, stretched out as far as they could in their harness. Cupid pulled in slack from each Reindeer's traces. I could hear the groan of the leather as they stretched even further outward.

Cupid gave a final jerk to Dasher's harness and then slipped back into her own traces, where Santa quickly tightened her harness and traces also. Almost before Santa hit the seat of the sleigh, we were off, climbing high into the snowy night sky.

Santa turned to me and explained, "A condition 3 is an emergency of the highest priority. It involves a human life. In this case, it's a busload of children high on a peak in Austria. The bus has slid off the high road and is dangling over the edge. The authorities are at a loss as to how to pull the bus back onto the slippery, icy road without dislodging it. If they fall, it's 13,000 feet down!"

I was scared stiff! What could we do? What could *I* do? Santa beckoned to me with his arm, his eyes still on the night sky in front of us. "Under your side of the seat, a box—get it quickly!"

I dropped to the floorboard as quickly as a cat and lifted up the double seat of the sleigh. I dropped the seat back down and put the box on top.

Glancing at me briefly, Santa said, "Now open it and you'll find a special breathing mask for each Reindeer. They're labeled with their names. I haven't time to fully explain, but I want you to fasten each mask over the nose and muzzle of each Reindeer. The small cylinder attached to each mask must be opened to the full position. It's a special mixture of stardust. It will enable them to breathe easier at the high altitude we must climb to without much exertion. They must save their strength for what we have to do."

I quickly grabbed a mask and discovered that it was Vixen's. She was halfway up the team. I had to clear my mind, to think straight. They were depending on me. I soon began to sort out the masks in the order in which the Reindeer were positioned.

On each mask, I checked the bottle and turned the valve to "full." I hooked the entire lot of masks into my belt and turned around, ready.

Santa quickly glanced at me and yelled, "GO!"

I cannot remember why I didn't hesitate when I jumped for Dasher's back. I do remember that all I could think about was those children in serious danger high on the mountain. Each Reindeer had not hesitated in the slightest at Santa's command.

It was all in order. I was a part of their team now; and so I jumped for all I was worth. I hit Dasher square in the middle of his broad back and held on for a split second. Clamping my legs around his middle, I whipped his stardust mask off my belt and swung it over his antlers. He lowered his head for me ever so slightly, but kept up the steady, driving rhythm that Blitzen had set for them. I slid the mask over his nose and hooked the back buckle tight.

Riding astride of Dasher's back, I looked at Cupid, who would be next.

I tried to measure the rhythm of their pounding hooves. When the time seemed right, I flung myself into space and found Cupid's soft fur. Clutching desperately, I righted myself onto her back. I brought the breathing mask over her nose and tightened the back buckle. *Two down*, I thought, *six to go*. The next jump would be difficult.

I was crisscrossing from side teams to side teams. Dancer quickly turned his head toward me. At his nod, I jumped again. A shift in the wind-turbulence brought me down hard on his back. He buckled at the knees a little. A heartbeat later, he was again driving hard with his legs to make up the lost step in rhythm.

I snatched the mask over his nose and adjusted the

buckle. We were climbing now, fast and high. I was beginning to struggle for air in these high altitudes.

After fitting masks on Prancer, Comet, and Vixen, I quickly looked at Grandfather Blitzen. What I saw scared me. His flanks were covered in white foam. The old Reindeer struggled for every breath in the icy coldness of height. His mouth was wide open, and I could hear the hoarseness coming from his lungs as he gasped for air.

He never slowed, but continued even harder the driving pace he had set. At that instant, that moment, I was terribly afraid for him. He wasn't going to make it! Two high climbs in one night were going to be too much... I got ready to jump for Blitzen, mask in hand. Donder could wait. He was much younger.

As I sprung for Blitzen's back, he shifted. Not much, but enough that I landed on Donder's back instead. With an awful cry, Blitzen screamed, never breaking his stride, *"Donder first!"*

In the split second that it took me to hook Donder's star mask onto him, I thought, of course, Blitzen would see to his team first, as a captain would be the last to leave a sinking ship.

Cupid's words rang in my ears: "And that's why he is the Grandfather... and why we love him so."

I sailed through space and threw my arms around his thick, massive neck. I would have to reach around his head. His antlers were much larger than those of the other Reindeer. I pushed myself up his neck and leaned to the inside of his harness. Besides this difficulty, Grandfather Blitzen must have been carrying close to 300 pounds of rope.

My only chance was to swing the mask around and hope to catch it with my left hand as the strap swung around his muzzle. 1–2–3, I let it go. I saw the strap disappear from sight, and I frantically felt for it with my left hand. *Got it!* With both hands, I leaned back and pulled the star mask down snug, and fastened the buckle behind his head.

With a sudden surge, Blitzen sprang forward, throwing me backwards along his back. The blue flames were coming off of his hooves like a welder's torch. His massive antlers were spraying me with brilliant stardust. I held onto Blitzen as we climbed even higher. We were in the Alps now!

Far ahead, I could just make out the red lights of the emergency vehicles. Closer, closer, we began to level out.

I could see the bus now! And I could hear the screams of frightened children. Each Reindeer could hear it too. The harness creaked and groaned as they stretched forward.

I was sure the leather bindings would snap from their efforts. I looked back at Santa, who was leaning forward, urging them on. I was still astride Blitzen when, through his star mask, he groaned, "The rope, get rid of the rope." I grabbed the draped coils of the heavy rope, and with all my strength I flung it to one side, away from us. The wind caught it, and it was quickly whipped backward, and immediately disappeared. Blitzen, relieved of the heavy load, flashed a sideways look at Donder. "Follow my lead, Donder, follow my lead."

Donder nodded and watched Blitzen out of the corner of one eye.

The bus was less than half a mile away as Blitzen started slowing the team. He was headed straight for the front of the bus.

Donder had grasped what Blitzen meant to do and began shouting orders back down the line. The other Reindeer understood clearly what Donder was saying. They began to brake under the direction of Vixen, who had thrust her front legs straight out in front of her. Comet had taken the same position. His hooves were straight out in front of him also.

The others began a backward motion with their legs, and just when it looked as though we would ram head-on into the bus, we slowly came to a gentle stop. Blitzen and Donder had their antlers set securely against the front grill of the bus.

The backward flurry of leg motion from the other Reindeer was keeping the sleigh in a stationary position. We hovered in midair, 13,000 feet up.

"*Now!*" ordered Blitzen.

Donder began to push with all his might, matching push for push with that of Grandfather Blitzen. Their back hooves were striking the outstretched front hooves of Comet and Vixen, who had kept their front legs extended forward.

I saw what they were doing in an instant! There was no traction in midair to push anything. Donder and Blitzen were using the front hooves of Comet and Vixen to gain their traction. Pushing in midair was a lot different from pulling in midair, I found out later.

As their hooves struck the hooves behind them, the entire team and sleigh was showered by sparkling cascades of stardust that soon had lit up the entire area.

The rescue teams had backed away when they saw us approach, but they had now come closer and were cheering the two struggling Reindeer on.

When hoof met hoof, it sounded like the clanging

of a blacksmith shop pounding iron against iron. The bus started to move slowly backwards, toward the safety of the road. Blitzen began driving even harder against the hooves of Comet, which were already starting to glow a warm red.

Donder gave a groan and drove harder. Vixen's hooves were taking a terrible beating from the back feet of Donder, but she held her position. Her hooves, too, were beginning to glow red from the friction.

I suddenly had an idea. I shouted to the rescuers standing on the road and asked if they had any water in their tank trucks. One of the men yelled back that they did. Trying to make myself heard over the tremendous clanging of their hooves, I told him to aim the water hose at the front feet of the second Reindeers.

"Cool them off!" I screamed, and pointed to the red-hot glow of their hooves.

Two of the men ran for the truck that held the water tanks. The other Reindeer were shifting their hovering motion, as they felt Donder and Blitzen gain ground. The entire team inched forward a little at a time. A cold jet-stream of water was sprayed from the tank and bathed the hooves of Comet and Vixen. I saw the red-hot glow go dull in color as the cold water did its work.

Blitzen and Donder, with a mighty groan, pushed the bus back onto the road safely. A hearty cheer went up from the rescue teams.

We didn't land, but went slowly past the bus to check on the welfare of the children. One child even leaned out of her window and gave Blitzen a quick hug. We circled the highest Alps and Santa steered them to a clearing, away from prying eyes, and landed.

We touched down and I heard the snow sizzle from the heat of Comet and Vixen's hooves. I jumped from Blitzen's back and fell to the soft, cold snow. I had been so filled with anxiety that I momentarily collapsed. Clearing my head, my first thought was to help Vixen and Comet.

I could hear Vixen whimpering from the pain. Comet was making a valiant effort not to cry. His head hung to the snow, his whole body trembling. Santa had jumped from the sleigh and was pulling a first-aid box from the back of the sleigh.

Blitzen and Donder had unhooked their traces and were shoveling snow over the front hooves of Comet and Vixen. The steam came through the cold snow in clouds. Santa came running up with the first-aid box and knelt quickly down beside the two Reindeer. Gently, he lifted one of Vixen's hooves from the packed snow and slowly examined it. After what seemed like a very long minute, Santa looked up and said, "Hoof burn. Painful, but not serious. It will heal in two or three days."

Santa spread some kind of ointment on each hoof. While he dressed the Reindeers' hooves, he talked to them softly. "Oh, my wonderful children, my precious children. You saved them. Not a thought for yourselves. You were magnificent."

Santa hugged them both and ordered a 15-minute stopover and said that they should remain standing in cold-packed snow. Blitzen and Donder immediately packed the cold snow around their hooves and stood by them, supporting them against the high winds of the Alps.

I went back to the sleigh with Santa and helped him pack the first-aid box away.

An Emergency of Highest Priority

Turning to me, Santa said, "Lad, never have I seen such a remarkable display of jumping. I never doubted that you could do it—even at such height and speed. You saved those children as much as my Reindeer did. Without their star masks, they wouldn't have had the strength to do what they did."

I shrugged, trying to put off his praise.

"Now, don't be modest. I'm going to move Comet and Vixen back a little and let Dancer and Prancer take their positions. It will be easier on their feet for the rest of the journey."

I had almost forgotten! It was Christmas Eve! We still had deliveries to make.

Sometime later, everyone was in fine spirits again, and talking about the emergency rescue. Comet and Vixen smiled modestly. They were still in some pain, but not so much that they didn't praise Blitzen and Donder for their magnificent display of strength.

Finally, Santa stepped forward and pinned a shiny gold medal for "valiant service" to Comet's and Vixen's shoulder harnesses. Everyone grew quiet.

Blitzen spoke up, too: "A fine pair of Reindeer you are. Aye! I'm so proud of both of you!"

All the Reindeer gathered around and congratulated Comet and Vixen. I was the last to approach them. "My words will tell of your deeds, and show the love that I hold for you both," I said with emotion.

Santa put his arm around my shoulder and nodded his approval.

As we started back to the sleigh, I heard Donder yell, "DUCK!" The cold, Austrian snowball exploded in my face. I turned to see Dancer looking at the clear night sky and whistling.

Wiping the snow from my face, I started laughing.

The seriousness of the moment had been broken. The others began to laugh, and we were all light-hearted once again, jolly and spirited.

Walking over to Dancer, I knelt down beside him. He was still looking up into the night sky. I whispered to him, "I'll get you back for that! Just wait!"

I walked back to the sleigh with a jump in my step. Dancer looked at me curiously, maybe even a bit worried.

As we climbed into the night sky, star masks and equipment safely tucked away under the seat again, I heard Santa boom, *"Away, Blitzen! Away!"* We continued on our Christmas Eve flight.

7

A Homecoming for Dancer and Prancer

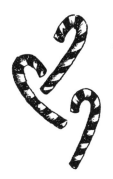

We traveled west through Switzerland at a dizzying speed, south into Italy, and then north into France. The list of goodies that Santa consumed was growing very long indeed. I had noticed that the toy bag was becoming considerably smaller and lighter, too. It seemed as though Santa did not grunt as loudly when he swung the bag free from the sleigh. All of us were quite tired.

I heard Dasher remark, "Good thing we're on the last leg. Mine are just about done in." Every Reindeer nodded.

My hand was aching because of all the writing I had done—and the difficulty of writing while we were moving through the air. I learned from Donder during a brief stopover in Paris that our route would take us next into Belgium, Holland, and then Denmark. Prancer and Dancer started showing signs of a little more life than usual, as we neared the border of Holland.

Santa leaned toward me, and pointing to the far north, said, "That's their homeland—Dancer and Prancer's. Each year in their hometown, the people celebrate the 'Festival of the Reindeer,' in which Dancer and Prancer are honored. It is a small village, where the only party they have, except for Christmas, is on the birthdays of Dancer and Prancer.

"They hold those two in great honor for having been chosen to be on my team. Let's see... it would have been in about 838 A.D. when they joined us. The people have never forgotten, and the story has been passed on for generations. It was a most magical night when they saw those two lift themselves up on the wind-currents and fly north along with Blitzen! You must be sure to ask Blitzen the whole story so that you can include it in your writings."

Dancer and Prancer were full of excitement now, and were actually tugging on their harnesses, irritating Blitzen a bit. He turned and stared hard at Dancer for a moment.

Santa turned the sleigh toward a small clearing just below us and brought the Reindeer down gently on the snow of the Netherlands.

Dancer and Prancer anxiously pawed the ground and mumbled excitedly between themselves. Cupid slipped her traces and deftly began to unhook Dancer and Prancer, who almost bounded to the front of the team, as the last hook that held them in place was unclipped.

Blitzen and Donder had already slipped their traces and moved back to take Dancer and Prancer's place. While Cupid hooked Dancer and Prancer into the two lead positions of the team, Santa finished hooking Donder and Blitzen into Dancer and Prancer's position.

If you weren't familiar with the positions of each Reindeer, their names and positions could become quite confusing. Santa got back into the sleigh and

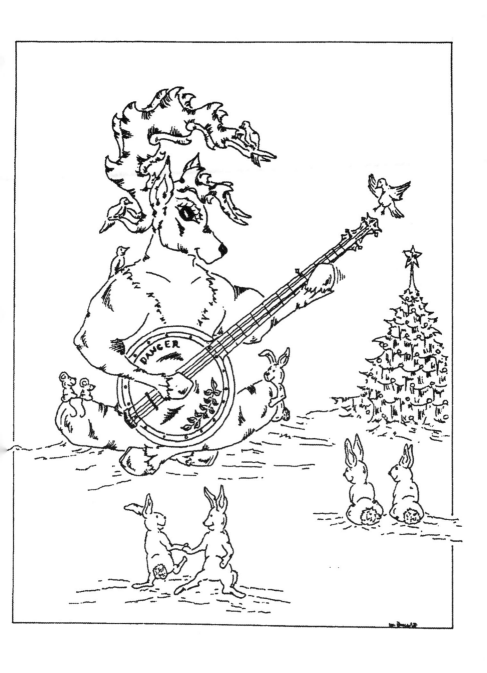

waited while Cupid shouldered her harness straps and fastened them tightly. She turned to Santa and nodded.

"*Away, Dancer... Away!*" boomed Santa.

I was very much in the dark as to what was going on. The sleigh was jerking and shaking badly due to Dancer's leading; and Prancer was having a difficult time trying to keep in step with Dancer. They both seemed very eager as they cleared the treetops and headed for the small village some five or six miles ahead.

For the lateness of the hour, the village certainly seemed to be awake. Lights beamed, especially around the tiny square, where it seemed a lot of activity was going on. I turned curiously to Santa.

Santa grinned and said, "The Village of Medemblik, their hometown. We always let them lead the sleigh and team into it every Christmas Eve. It's become a tradition for them."

The two new lead Reindeer were straining at the harness, trying to proceed faster toward the village. Because Blitzen and Donder were somewhat larger than Dancer and Prancer, their traces hung around the smaller Reindeers' shoulders loosely. Dancer's almost sagged. Yet they pressed on.

A short, barking order from Blitzen caused me to look at Dancer. "Step lively, Dancer, or you'll lose the traces! To the right, now, Prancer... stay with Dancer. Aye, that's the ticket. A little slower. We want to get there in one piece!"

Dancer had lost his footing and was starting to slump backwards in Blitzen's traces. Donder moved up quickly. Placing one hoof under Dancer's rump, he gave him a quick shove upright, which caused Dancer to level out evenly.

We swept into the village square, where about 300 townspeople, perhaps the entire population of this small village, had gathered to welcome their beloved Reindeer home once again.

Prancer held his head high, and Dancer was certainly stepping high when we circled the square and came down next to a very large water fountain. The two lead Reindeer were dancing and prancing and shaking their antlers to throw off showers of sparkling stardust.

We took in the "Welcome Home!" signs, enjoyed the hot refreshments, and collected more gifts. I couldn't understand the language of the people, but we saw how Dancer and Prancer were greatly loved. They were received warmly and enthusiastically, with many hugs and pats from children and grownups alike. Then, after a short welcoming speech from the mayor, who presented Santa with the key to the city, we took off once again.

As I looked back, I saw that the town square was virtually deserted. In fact, I could see no one. I looked, puzzled, at Santa.

"It's Christmas Eve, Lad," laughed Santa. "They have gone to their beds, lest Santa Claus pass them by."

Of course, Santa couldn't deliver the toys and presents if the town were awake. We circled the town for some 15 minutes, having returned the Reindeer to their rightful places in the harness. Dancer and Prancer didn't mind. They were grateful, realizing that everyone had joined in to make their homecoming terrific. They gazed affectionately at the others and were content.

I, however, was starting to become quite excited.

We were coming up on Norway, having cleared the North Sea. After Norway, I knew we would be headed straight home. The North Pole! The place I had dreamed about as a boy. I was going to see what dreams were made of! And I would learn how each Christmas Reindeer had come to that special place. I was so anxious that I choked on a cup of hot chocolate I had brought with me from Medemblik!

Santa thumped me on the back, and, after looking at me hard, asked, "How would you like to help me make some deliveries in Norway, Lad?"

"Would I? Do candy canes have stripes? Do Reindeer fly? Does Santa have a white beard?" (Actually, it was silver!)

Santa laughed, then replied, "Get ready with the toy sack, Lad. Our first stop is just here." He pointed down.

We landed atop an elegant Nordic home, complete with decorative trim. As I shouldered the toy sack and started for the chimney, I heard Dancer say, "His first chimney! This should be good!" I eagerly jumped to the chimney and was just about to plummet down when Santa grabbed me.

"Whoa, Lad, whoa! This is how it's done," Santa said.

There was a flash of light, and I found myself standing beside Santa in the living room of the home. Santa quickly took the toy sack and began pulling presents from it, placing these around the Christmas tree. I watched, spellbound, as he went straight to his work. Finally, with a sweep of his red-robed arm, he trimmed the Christmas tree with Christmas spirit. The tree came alive for an instant and twinkled brightly as this special gift swept through its green branches.

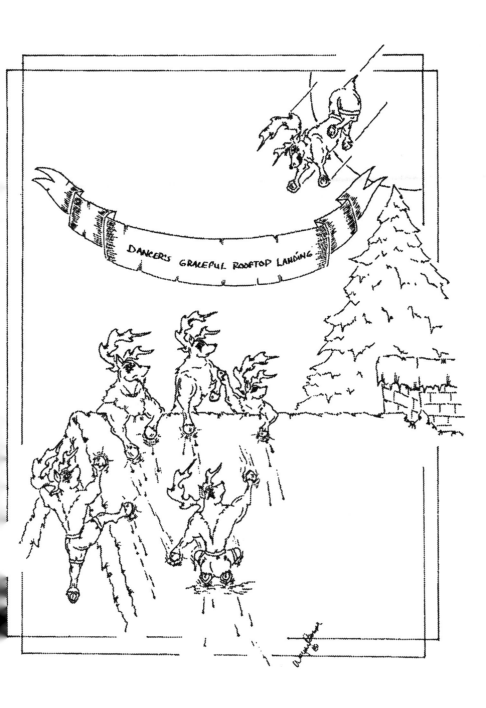

Standing back to survey his work, Santa glanced over at the plateful of sandwiches and the hot chocolate that had been left out for him. I winked at him. "It'll be our secret this time!"

"She knows already, Lad," Santa said, laughing. "She's already writing it down." Santa offered me a sandwich from the plate and whispered, "Shall we?"

When we had finished, we looked at each other guiltily, and then burst out laughing. "Now you can write about the night you supped with ol' Claus in Norway, eh, Lad?"

Back on the rooftop, I excitedly told the Reindeer about my visit. They listened politely, smiles on their faces. Little did I know that each Reindeer had many times made such indoor visits with the good Santa Claus.

I told them about what I had seen, what I had felt, and how my heart had pounded so, seeing the Christmas tree lit up with Christmas spirit. It was a visit I would remember all my life!

Santa stood up and stretched, took a deep breath, and patted his stomach. Smiling, he said, "Let's go! There are many stops yet, and then home!"

I was allowed to make many more visits down below, as the Reindeer called it. And each time I was even more amazed.

We traveled with great intent now. We were almost through with our magical journey. I found myself wishing we were through so that Blitzen and Donder could turn the sleigh north, toward the great star that was ever present off to our left.

The Reindeer were anxious also, but they never let this rush them in the performance of their tasks. Every child had to be taken care of before we could return.

Santa paused every now and then to check his maps, making sure he had covered all the territory. After what seemed like hours, Santa announced that the last village was Hammerfest. It was just off the coast of the Barents Sea.

We made our deliveries in Hammerfest, and as Santa disappeared down the last chimney, I took a moment to gaze at the star that held the secret of home. The North Pole would be our next stop! The Reindeer gazed at it too. Dasher pawed at the fresh snow atop the roof.

Remember, all during our trip, I had written down what Cupid had told me Santa had eaten. There was a stack of notepads filled with my writings. Another stack held notes containing my experiences during the flights. All of these papers were in the back of the sleigh, which looked empty now that all the toys had been delivered. I almost felt let down at seeing the emptiness of that toy compartment.

Donder came back and sensed my feelings. "Don't grieve, Lad," he said. "This feeling will last but a little time, and then it will pass. Santa will check his list twice to make doubly sure that no child was missed tonight. When he's sure, then we'll head for home. Watch the star, Lad. You'll be caught up in Christmas as we draw even closer to the great star. The magic is strongest there—you'll know it with all your heart and soul."

Prancer, who never had a lot to say, nudged my arm. "There's much more once we get home! You'll have plenty to keep you busy. And don't forget, *tomorrow's Christmas morning!*"

Suddenly, a chorus of "Merry Christmas!" filled the air, as the Reindeer in turn wished each other—and me—the merriest Christmas ever.

"A Merry Christmas to all of you," boomed Santa, who had returned to the rooftop. In his hand was a brightly wrapped package. He motioned for us to gather around him. We made a semicircle around Santa, and he put the present down in front of Comet and Vixen.

"This present," Santa said, "was addressed to all of you by the two children who live here. It is a very special present, I think." There was a shiny twinkle in Santa's eye. "Comet, Vixen, our two gold heart recipients—the two children would approve, I'm sure, that you two should be the ones to open it—for all the Reindeer."

As Comet held the package, Vixen deftly pulled the bright paper from it and lifted the lid. There were small sighs from each Reindeer as they saw the contents. It was a small, wooden Nativity scene, carved and painted by the two children. It must have taken them many hours to complete. The tag that the package bore simply stated, "To all of you. We love you."

We were all silent for a moment. Then, Cupid spoke very softly, hardly above a Reindeer whisper. "And that's what Christmas is all about."

The Reindeer asked if I would hold the Nativity scene for them until we reached home. There, it would be properly displayed on the main mantel in the Great Hall of Toys.

I clutched the box tightly as Santa gently raised the reins. He looked at me and then, with a smile, shouted: *"Happy Christmas to all, and to all a good night!"*

Soon we were airborne, headed for the North Pole! There was urgency in each step. The Christmas Reindeer were pulling toward the Great Star. Their antlers began to glow a sparkling gold as they drew nearer the magical beams of the star. Their hooves grew in color to a brilliant blue, twinkling with glittery stardust. The star even seemed to glow brighter as if to welcome us all back after our long journey.

I felt extremely tired, but exhilarated. I had my list to give to Mrs. Claus. I had the notes I had taken on the journey. And I knew I had my work cut out for me after I arrived.

As I thought about what I would do first, I heard Donder, from 'way up front, yell, *"Duck, Lad!"* The cold snowball hit me squarely in the face and exploded around my head. I wiped the soft mush off and heard the hysterical laughter from all of them, even Santa, who was thumping me on the back. Quickly, I looked toward Dancer. He was laughing so hard he was doubled up in the harness, simply being dragged along by the rest of them.

He stopped laughing just long enough to sputter, "That's Norwegian snow, Lad. Ain't it cold?" He was laughing so hard then, that he draped one arm over Prancer to hold himself in the harness. I began to laugh.

I laughed so hard, I fell off the seat and crumpled onto the floor of the sleigh, slapping my hand on the sleigh seat. We were still laughing as we passed through the magical beams of the Great Star and were bathed in the warmth of its rays. We were still chuckling when Santa turned the sleigh and we descended.

We landed in front of the Great Hall of Toys, where we were greeted by hundreds of cheering elves and Mrs. Claus, who held out a tray of steaming mugs filled with hot chocolate for all of us. We were home!

8

A Christmas Eve Party —North Pole Style

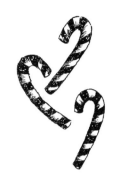

A crowd soon gathered around the sleigh and Reindeer with shouts of, "Welcome home! Welcome home!"

Several elves ran forward to unhook the Reindeer, and began to neatly fold the harness so that it could be stored until it was needed again. Santa and I stepped from the sleigh into a sea of elves.

Then Mrs. Claus came forward through the "sea" and hugged Santa tightly. She turned to me, smiling, and said, "Welcome to the North Pole, Lad." Then she hugged me tightly too. She continued, "Santa and I have talked about your coming for quite a long time now. We both felt the time was right that you should come and tell the Reindeer's stories. From the looks of all that paper in the sleigh, I think Santa has made a good decision."

I blushed, not knowing what to say. Finally I managed to stammer, "Thank you, Ma'am. It is an honor to be here. I hope to prove worthy of the task Santa has entrusted to me."

"Now," she said, smiling, "we must take care of our children and see that they are fed and warmed. Their backs must be rubbed with liniment, for I'm sure they're very tired." She began to supervise several elves, who were walking beside the Reindeer with soft curry combs, brushes, and blankets in their hands.

Santa touched me on the shoulder. "Stay with them, Lad. There has been a place prepared for you in their quarters. Very neatly done, too." I turned to hurry after the Reindeer as Santa called after me, "Don't tarry too long, any of you—for tonight's still Christmas Eve. Mrs. Claus and I will be in the Great Hall of Toys waiting."

I passed Mrs. Claus, who took Santa in hand. They entered their house—it was a charming, small stone castle. I could faintly hear her scolding as they went through the archway. "How could you have eaten so much? And after you assured me you would cut back, especially on the eggnog...!"

Donder looked up. "There'll be elf-madness to pay now for Santa. Cupid must have given Mrs. Claus the list."

Behind us, the elves were slowly pulling the sleigh toward a small, neat shed, where it would be kept until needed again. I suddenly thought of the blue star still in its bag under the front seat of the sleigh. Donder stopped me as I turned to go and retrieve it.

"We'll get it later when Blitzen is asleep." I nodded and fell into step beside Donder. We trudged through the snow up a small hill that overlooked Santa's home and workshop. When we topped a small rise we had been climbing, I stared in disbelief.

There in front of me was a very neat clearing ringed by evergreens. Scattered here and there in the clearing, and even into the evergreens, were eight of the quaintest cottages I had ever seen. Each Reindeer had his or her own home, and they had personally styled them—some were in the Nordic tradition, some in the Swiss, to fit their homeland origins.

"Well, I'll be..." I stammered.

"If people think I'm going to lie on a pile of dirty straw and hay at night, they don't know me very well," said Donder. "Our houses are basically like yours. Each piece of furniture was designed by us, made by the elves. Much better than some old stable! A good thing, too, as you're bunking with me!"

I hesitated. "Are you sure, Donder? I don't want to put you out."

"Actually, I requested it. We certainly couldn't put you in with Blitzen! He's too set in his ways. Since I'm second-lead Reindeer, it was logical. Besides, I really do want your company, and I can help fill in more details for your writing."

Donder's living room had a beautiful Christmas tree set beside a glowing fireplace. The walls were decorated with pictures of the team in Christmases past, and with many pictures of small children. A throw-rug in the middle of the floor had a beautiful snow scene woven into the fabric. And next to the fireplace was a trophy case holding Donder's awards.

"It's beautiful, Donder. I love it!"

Donder let out a small breath of air. "Good!" He motioned for me to sit down in a comfortable easy chair. Then he disappeared.

He returned almost immediately, carrying two steaming mugs. "Hot chocolate, North Pole style," he said, and handed me a mug. The handle was shaped like Reindeer antlers and the mug looked like a snowball with silver glitter all over it.

Donder had slipped his starshoes off and donned

a comfortable-looking pair of woolly slippers that resembled Christmas stockings. He collapsed in another chair and murmured, "*Ahhhh.*"

After some light conversation, I felt so warm and relaxed that I must have dozed off. Who knows how much later, I was awakened by Donder's nudging my shoulder gently.

"Hey, come on. We've got to get over to the Great Hall of Toys for the Christmas Eve celebration. Here is your room," he pointed it out. "You'll find some fresh clothes..."

I found pants, something like knickers, and I chuckled as I put on red and white candy-cane-striped stockings. The shoes were, predictably, turned up at the toes. A bright red shirt and green vest completed the outfit.

As we left Donder's house, we were joined by Cupid and Dasher. "You look magnificent," said Cupid, looking at me with her big brown eyes.

A little farther on we were joined by Comet and Vixen, still limping somewhat, but both refreshed and ready for the big celebration.

The Great Hall of Toys was enormous! In fact, from the front door where we entered, I could not see to the end of it.

Donder pushed me on inside, where hundreds of elves—dressed much as I was—were milling around, laughing and singing. Donder guided me over to the left door as other Reindeer came through.

The colors and sparkles were overwhelming. From the high ceilings hung branches of sweet-smelling, living greens, complete with holly berries.

Donder told me that the population of the North Pole was approximately 653. Each elf was a specialist

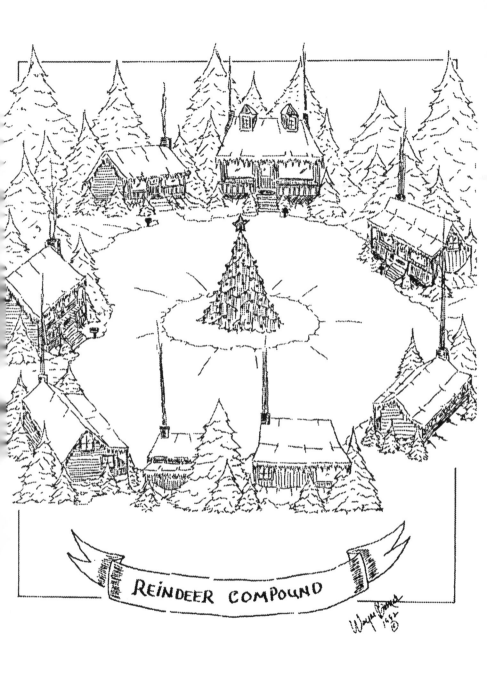

in some area: toy-making, building, tailoring, cooking, any skill needed. Some of the elves specialized in Reindeer care: hooves, skin, antlers.

We slowly moved through the crowd of elves toward the center of the room, where Santa and Mrs. Claus had set up a long table of refreshments. Santa was laughing; and several of the other Reindeer were there: Dasher and Cupid beside Mrs. Claus, and Blitzen beside Santa. They were reminiscing about the night's adventures.

Mrs. Claus was very stout, like her husband. And she had the most remarkably kind face. There was not a wrinkle in her skin, and she smiled sweetly most of the time. She reminded me of all the grandmothers of the world in one person. She wore a splendid hoop skirt of apple red. Fine white lace adorned the dress, and in her hair of silver she wore a golden comb. Her eyes sparkled like diamonds. And her rosy cheeks were complemented by very high, soft eyebrows.

She steered me toward an array of delectable-looking dishes, and heaped my plate full of Christmas treats. As we got to know each other, I asked her if Santa was very angry about the list of what he had eaten—the one that Cupid and I had compiled during our flight.

Smiling, she said, "Oh, he acts put out. But he knows it is all because we care about him."

All around the Great Hall were Christmas trees that had been decorated in styles from all over the world. An enormous fireplace, 10 feet wide and 10 feet high, threw out a warm blaze as elves kept logs piled high on it.

The Reindeer played games such as "Push the Reindeer," in which someone would grab the Reindeer's antlers and try to push him backwards. This led to contests of strength, and much shouting and playful fun.

After awhile, when the laughter of good conversation and games had subsided, Santa took his fork and hit the side of his glass several times until he had the attention of the entire party. "Another Christmas Eve journey has been completed, and with great success," he began. "I would like to thank the fine Christmas Reindeer who pulled their load faithfully once again for another year."

Everyone clapped and applauded heartily, toasting the Reindeer with their punch. Then he said, "I would also like to call to everyone's attention to the fine young man we have returned with." I began to blush. I didn't know this was on the agenda.

"This fine friend is going to write the story of our Christmas Reindeer and how they came to pull our sleigh. We wish him all good fortune, and will give him whatever assistance he needs. From the looks of what he has already written, I don't think he's going to have much trouble!"

Next, as Mrs. Claus joined him, he beckoned to three elves, who came forth bearing three beautifully engraved wooden boxes, decorated with Reindeer motifs.

"Tonight," said Santa, "as we journeyed over the world to complete our mission, we were once again rewarded by knowing that we had brought much happiness to the children of the world." Then he told all at the party in detail of the rescue of the children in the Alps, and the loyalty and courage of the marvelous Christmas Reindeer.

By the time he had finished, Mrs. Claus was wiping her eyes gently with a handkerchief, and the elves had lowered their heads in respect.

Santa scanned the crowd and said, "Will Comet and Vixen come forward, please?" The way parted, and the two Reindeer walked up side by side. Mrs. Claus opened two of the small wooden boxes she had placed on the table, and from each she drew forth a sparkling chain of gold with a single heart attached to it.

She deftly leaned forward and placed these chains around the necks of Comet and Vixen, kissing each on the side of the muzzle. There was great cheering, and the crowd gathered up to hug and congratulate them.

Santa quieted everyone again, and announced: "We are indeed proud of Comet and Vixen. The Great Ledger of Deeds will record tonight that they both received the 'Gold Heart' award for valiant service to the children of the world." The applause was deafening.

Finally Santa had to tap his glass again. "Quiet, please! We have one more recognition to make." The elves hushed and everyone turned toward Santa.

"Tonight, during our condition 3, a very brave action was performed by Lad here. He, without hesitation, played the most daring game of leapfrog *during flight*, from one Reindeer's back to the next, at very high altitudes, to place the star masks on each Reindeer. For our success, we must thank him also!"

There was a loud gasp, and I suddenly understood that I had done something either pretty stupid—or incredibly daring.

Santa motioned for me to stand in front of him. Mrs. Claus picked up the last wooden box and handed it to him. Presenting me the box, Santa said, "For

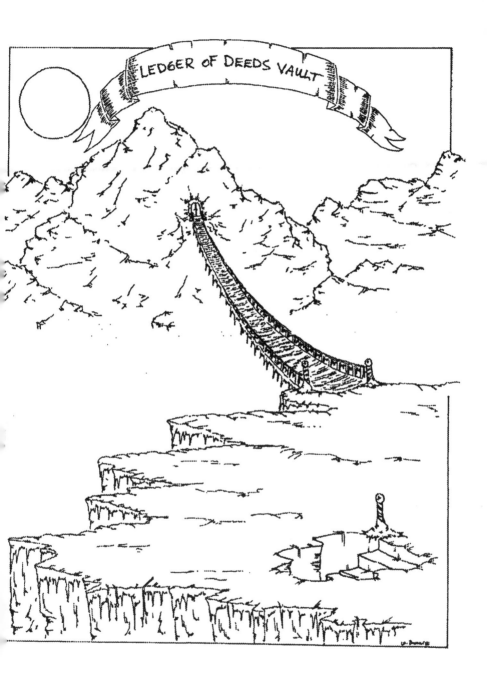

valiant performance and without question, the Reindeer of Christmas and I are very proud to award to you the Medal of Christmas Eve. Your deed, too, will be recorded in the Great Ledger of Deeds as your first step toward the distinguished 'Silver Flight Medal!'"

Santa leaned forward and pinned a small golden Christmas tree to the lapel of my vest, then shook my hand.

There were cheers; and elves thumped my back and cried, "*Hear! Hear!*"

Donder came up and put his arm around my shoulder and led me toward the table. "Now grab another piece of cake," he advised. "We've still got a few things left to do tonight. It's Christmas Eve, remember?"

I wasn't very hungry. I just wanted to look at and touch the medal they had given me—to be sure it was real!

Finally, we went to stand in the line that was gathering in front of Santa and Mrs. Claus, to say goodnight and Merry Christmas.

As we left the party, Donder whispered to me, "We've got to go retrieve that blue star if we want to get it into Grandfather Blitzen's stocking in time for Christmas morning!"

And so we made our way to the front of the Great Hall of Toys, saying our last Christmas Eve wishes to all we passed. And we stepped through the double doors into the cold, crisp air of the North Pole.

9

Christmas Magic and Donder's Story

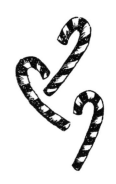

Donder and I paused for a moment and listened to the elf orchestra playing a medley of Christmas carols outside the doors of the Great Hall of Toys. It had started to snow very gently, and it seemed as if the evergreens were swaying to the music.

The brightly colored decorations outside were magnificent. Some of the elves had made snowmen, which sported top hats and black mittens. The whole scene was indeed a Christmas story come true!

We watched as Dasher and Comet made their way up the hill that led to their homes. Suddenly a bustling behind us caused us to turn and look back. At least ten elves were trying to put Grandfather Blitzen's topcoat on him before he walked up to his house. Of course, Blitzen was having none of it—yet even through his complaining, it was clear that the elves were winning. Finally they secured Blitzen's heavy plaid coat around his shoulders. The old Reindeer continued up the hill, mumbling to himself. We watched as he disappeared into the falling snow.

Donder pulled me aside. "You go and fetch the star, just yonder, in that shed where the sleigh is kept. I'll keep watch so no one sees you."

Quickly, I slipped around the side of the building and, feeling like a private detective, scurried quickly into the shed. The sleigh had been draped with a heavy material, and I could feel the heat coming off the runners. Faint stardust lit the interior of the shed, so no light was necessary. I pulled up the heavy draping and groped under the front seat for the star-bag. I pulled it out and lowered the draping to cover the sleigh again. I tiptoed to the door and peeped over.

Donder motioned for me to come out, as the coast was clear. "Follow me," he murmured.

We ran around the side of the Great Hall, and Donder anxiously peered around the corner. I saw what looked like Santa Claus sneak past us in the dark and head for the very shed I had just come out of. He disappeared. "Look!" whispered Donder, pointing to the evergreens on our left.

Turning, I saw Grandfather Blitzen gliding through the trees, a pack hanging from his antlers. Nudging Donder, I asked, puzzled, "What's going on here?"

He stifled a chuckle and said, "There's magic afoot every Christmas Eve. It's always the same. Everyone sneaks around trying to put presents in everyone else's stocking. Look here..."

I couldn't believe it. Mrs. Claus and several elves were busy lugging something up the hill to the Reindeer compound. Quickly, they would duck into a snowdrift whenever they thought someone was coming. We saw other Reindeer, as well, doing similar sneaking around.

Donder had a plan for us. "We'll circle the hill and come up from the back," he said, as we jumped a big snowdrift. It took a few minutes, but we finally made

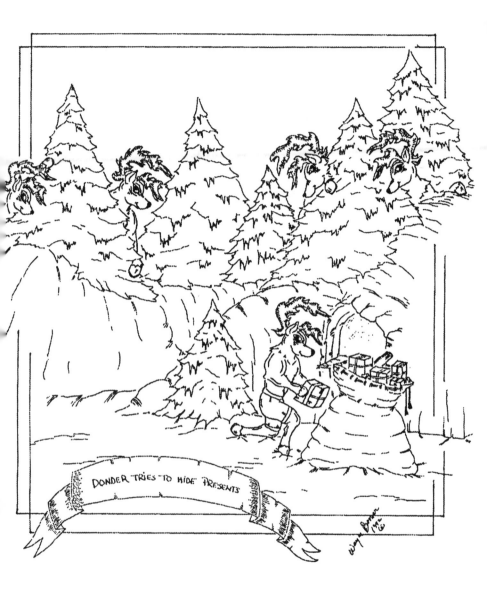

it to Blitzen's back door. Everything seemed quiet. He told me to hop on his back and grab his antlers. This I did, and he flew to the top of Blitzen's house, landing beside the chimney.

He took the star-bag and reached inside, grabbing the blue star we had caught while plunging through the Tropic of Capricorn. He pulled it out—never have I seen such a brilliant blue! Donder quickly stepped to the side of the chimney, and with all his might—the star raised above his antlers, clutched in his front hooves—he sent it plummeting down the chimney of Blitzen's house.

Almost immediately, a shower of blue and silver sparks issued from the chimney with such magnitude that I thought we had set fire to Blitzen's house! But Donder quickly explained that when the blue star had entered the house, it began to dissipate in all directions. The star was bathing everything in the house with its power. "Now we have given him enough star energy to last maybe... 500 years! It will make Grandfather Blitzen feel younger as he absorbs the energy around him. He's going to need it, after two high climbs tonight!"

Then we returned to Donder's house to pick up the bag of presents he had stashed away for the other Reindeer. We flew from house to house and delivered them all—though I felt bad about not having anything to give them myself. I found that it wasn't necessary to go down each chimney, as Donder simply threw the presents down. They magically found their own way to the Christmas stockings under each tree or hanging on a fireplace mantel.

Donder even threw a present down Santa's chimney. It was a beard warmer that could be worn to bed!

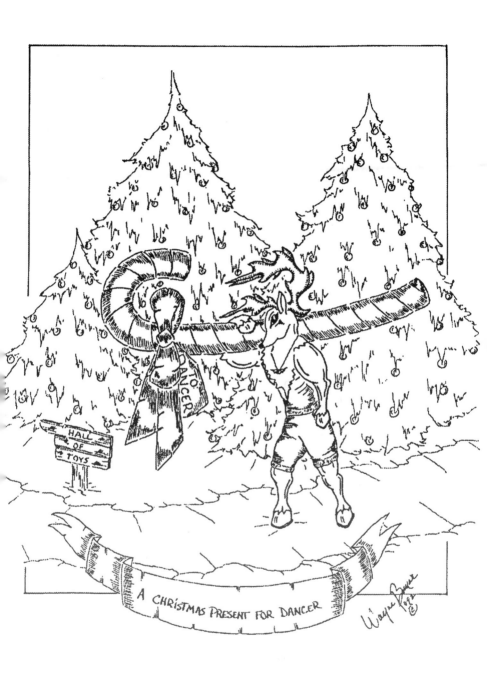

Around daybreak, as we were finishing our deliveries, we happened to run into Grandfather Blitzen! Startled, he stared at us, cleared his throat, and said, "'Tis very late for you two young bucks to be out and about. Aye, it is."

We didn't say anything, but just nodded respectfully. As far as we could tell, we and Grandfather Blitzen were the only ones still up. I was completely exhausted, but we had one more stop.

When we reached Dancer's chimney, I saw him drop in a large, heavy volume of something. "It's the complete set of 10,001 knock-knock jokes! He'll drive everyone crazy with them," Donder explained.

I asked if he had time for one more "delivery." He was puzzled, but watched closely as I gathered some flexible branches from a nearby evergreen tree. Donder sat on a snowdrift while I constructed a "snowball launcher" that would be released when Dancer opened his front door that morning. I hadn't forgotten his snowball pranks!

The principle of my device was simple. When the playful Reindeer opened his front door, the trigger consisting of a flexible branch would release a larger branch—holding a snowball roughly two feet in diameter! I had positioned it so that it was aimed at the front door, about the same height as Dancer's face.

I felt satisfied now. "If I weren't so tired, I'd knock on his door right now," I said. "I expect we'll hear him scream, though, all the way from our house!"

We returned to Donder's home, collapsed in our beds, and were soon fast asleep. I don't know how we managed to miss seeing the huge piles of gifts that had filled up Donder's living room in our absence! Clearly the others had successfully completed their Christmas deliveries, just as we had.

How long we slept, I can't say. I know that I dreamed of Christmas. When I awoke, I knew that not only Santa, but all his Reindeer, and their magic as well, had been at work.

Donder stirred from across the room, and I watched as he lifted one eyelid, then both. I asked if he was feeling the Christmas magic, too.

"I dreamed I was a fawn again," he said, smiling. That was almost 1,300 years ago. I was born in the Black Mountains of Denmark in the year 705 A.D.

"There is one Christmas morning I will never forget. I was one year old, and my mother roused me out of a sound sleep. She told me that Sinta Klauss had been there. As I sleepily teetered into the outer stable, my father picked me up and carried me to a small decorated Christmas tree that had been set up by the old farmer's son. It was aglow with shiny decorations as well as little carved wooden ornaments. I had never seen such a beautiful sight!

"Everything was different that morning. I remember there was sweet corn and oats for us, and I recall the friendship of all the animals. We gathered around the tree and my father handed me a small package wrapped in sparkling silver paper and tied with bright red ribbons.

"He told me that this was a special gift from the great Christmas Reindeer, Blitzen. I had heard that famous name—he was the one who pulled the magnificent sleigh of the good Sinta Klauss. I had often thought how wonderful it would be to travel through the skies with Sinta Klauss, to bring such happiness to all children—fawns included—on wonderful Christmas Eve night.

"As I opened the package, I felt shivers of great joy

and a wonderful sense of belonging run through me. Inside the package was a pair of hoof mittens that had been made by Mrs. Klauss. As I hurriedly put them on, my father bent over to pick up the letter that had fallen to one side. In my childish delight over the present, I had not seen the letter. My father read it silently, as the rest of our family watched. The paper was bordered in stardust. He handed it over to my mother and she read it out loud. At once, I stopped and listened.

"It said, 'My Dear Little One: It is with great anticipation and pleasure that I write to you this Christmas letter. The good Sinta Klauss and I have many more stops to make before morning dawns. We tarried here so that we might watch you in the night air as we watched you in sleep. For we have observed you for many days now, Little One.

"You have grown wonderfully and faithfully in your childhood, and soon you will be an adult. A time of responsibility now faces you. Your faith in us and Christmas has never faltered. You are strong in body and mind.

"The ways of the world are changing even now. The journey that I and the good Sinta Klauss make each Christmas Eve grows larger with each passing year. We have searched the world for such as you, Little One. The time has come when you must make a decision. Sinta Klauss and I have chosen you to help us on our journey each year. The choice of whether to accept our call is yours alone.

"Should you decide to journey with us, be ready to embark next Christmas Eve on an eternity of happiness and joy. But, know this, Little One, that with the passage of each year you will see and experience

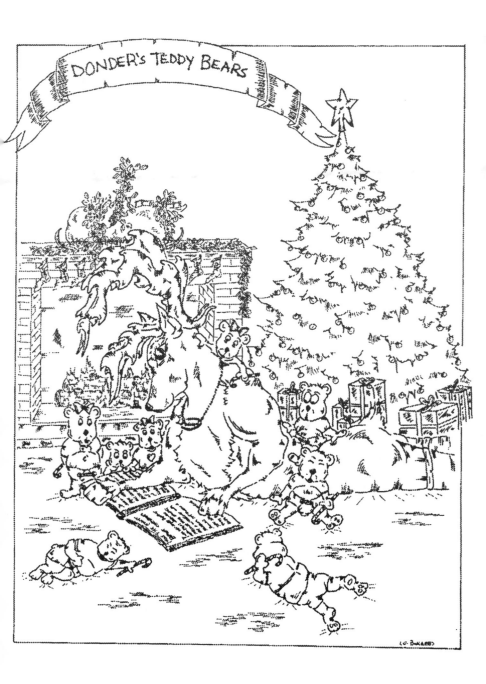

wondrous things. Your only reward will be the happiness in a child's face, and knowing that you have done well by your labors. So arise, little 'Donder,' for that will be your Christmas name if you decide to travel with us; for it means 'A Stout Puller of Faith.'"

Donder was silent for a moment. Then he continued, "It was signed, 'Blitzen, the first of many.' Although I was not quite grown, I understood his words. Of course, my parents cried. Not with grief, but with great joy! They understood that I had been chosen to help pull the magical sleigh—to immortality.

"It was a very special Christmas for me and my family, and throughout that year they urgently trained me in the ways of a good and responsible adult Reindeer. After another year had passed, I was a strong, young buck.

"I waited with my family outside on that Christmas Eve, and we searched the skies for the sleigh of the good Sinta Klauss. I was afraid. Afraid of leaving everything I had grown up with—my parents, my village.

"My father, seeing my anxiety, took me to one side. We stood together, overlooking our village all covered with snow. My father told me that this was not an ending, but a beginning—a beginning of something pure and wondrous. That I alone had been chosen to fly the magical wind-currents of time and help bring peace and joy to the world.

"He said that I was not to be afraid of the truth, and that he would be with me always. My father then leaned down and kissed me on the forehead. He had never done that before. I hugged him tightly, and as we stood in the snow, I felt his tears as they fell like raindrops.

"We turned at the sound of sleighbells, and saw the great first-chosen Christmas Reindeer standing there. The good Sinta Klauss hitched me into the harness beside the great Blitzen. We made ready to take off, all of our good-byes being said.

"Then my father put his hoof on my shoulder and said for all to hear, 'Pull well, my Stout Puller of Faith, for the young ones of the world will depend on you. I am very proud to call you my son, Great Donder!'

"As we climbed high into the night sky, my father grew smaller and smaller, until only a small speck remained on the ground. But I remember how tall and majestic he looked that night. I have carried his dignity, and my mother's love, with me since then."

It had been a time of immense sharing that Christmas morning as Donder told me the story of his call from Santa. I asked him only one question concerning that Christmas Eve of so long ago: "Were there any regrets?"

Donder smiled and looked thoughtful as he gave his reply. "No regrets, Lad. It has been just as my father said it would be. Great truth and beauty. Through all the adventures I have had, and those yet to come, I know my father is with me—always."

Smiling at each other, we turned again to the contents of the present-packed living room. Donder said, "Well, it seems that Santa Claus has been here, along with many of his helpers."

Then he let out a howl and dove into a pile of gaily wrapped packages, yelling, *"Come on! Let's open our Christmas presents!"*

10

Christmas Breakfast with Santa and Blitzen's Story of Love

After opening all of our presents, we once again had Donder's living room looking neat and clean. Once all the paper had been picked up, Donder stretched his forelegs and, giving a little kick with his back legs, said, "We'd better hurry and go get properly dressed. We have a Christmas morning engagement to attend to. Santa and Mrs. Claus always have us over to their house for early Christmas Breakfast."

This thought really got me moving fast: Christmas with Santa!

I was all thumbs in my excitement. Donder watched with amusement as I nearly tore my new shirt putting it on backwards. I clumsily pulled on my new shoes that Comet and Dasher had given me, and placed my new compass—which was my present from Grandfather Blitzen—in my shirt pocket.

Donder put on his new topcoat given to him by Santa and Mrs. Claus, and his new mittens from Vixen and Cupid. "Ready?" he asked.

Was I ever! I held the door for Donder as we stepped out into the gently falling snow and started across the white-encrusted compound. I stopped for a moment beside the tall Christmas tree, looking up to the very top at its shining star, and said a silent prayer of thanks, wishing our Lord a Happy Birthday. Donder was just lifting his head from prayer also when we both said, "Amen." Then we added, shouting at the sky, "Merry Christmas, world!"

We began to trot down the hill, our hearts full of Christmas spirit. Just as we reached the front walk of Santa's house, we heard someone shouting, "Hey, wait up. *Wait a minute!*"

We turned and saw Dancer running down the hill. I thought I could see snow still clinging to his antlers from the snowball trap I had set up in front of his door. He came panting up, his breath making small clouds of frosty smoke. He held out a small Christmas present for me.

"We're even now, Lad! No hard feelings, OK? It was all in the Christmas spirit," said Dancer.

"Go ahead, open the present," said Donder.

I smiled, and Dancer grinned further as I pulled at the paper. I turned to Donder and held it away from myself, while it was still partially wrapped. "Here, if you're so sure, *you* open it!" I said to Donder.

"No way! It's your present," he insisted.

Feeling doubtful, I opened the package very slowly. Inside was the ugliest hat I have ever seen. First, it had ear flaps—which I hate. And it was pointed on top—with a fluffy green ball of fuzz adorning its topmost point. I could just hear the kidding I would get for wearing it. "Oh, his hat fits his head—same shape." If I wore this "present," I would look like a deranged Martian with a gigantic green ball on his head! "Uh, thanks, Dancer," I said dubiously.

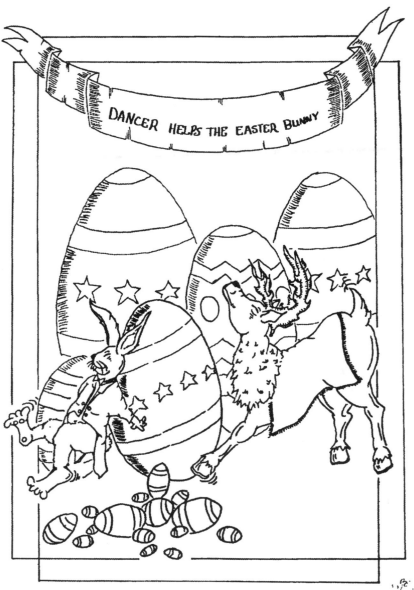

Dancer was laughing so hard I thought he was going to fall over.

After he had pulled himself together, and I had stuck the hat under my arm—hoping I wouldn't be asked about it at the breakfast—we continued on to Santa's.

It was warm and cozy inside the Clauses' hallway. The first thing I noticed was the huge hatrack inside the door, on which hung Santa's great red robe and hat. His big, black boots stood nearby on the floor. Santa himself took our coats and hung them next to his.

Then he hurried us into the living room, where several of the other Christmas Reindeer were sitting, talking with Mrs. Claus. He told us to make ourselves at home and help ourselves to the hot chocolate on the side table.

I was greatly impressed with the beauty of the room. Everywhere were branches of evergreens, hung from the massive wooden beams that ran the length of the ceiling. The tinsel and decorations on them sparkled and glittered as the firelight danced off each one.

An enormous chandelier hung from the center of the room, turning around ever so slightly. It sparkled with light in all colors of the rainbow. The brightly polished walls were covered with portraits of all the Christmas Reindeer, some wearing their many medals and awards, some standing with Santa Claus. There was one picture of Mrs. Claus bottle-feeding a very small Reindeer.

"That's Cupid," Santa interrupted my thoughts as I gazed at this picture. "It's just after Blitzen brought her to us as a little one. Mrs. Claus was like a mother to her, always feeding her and taking her for walks.

For several years, Cupid wouldn't eat unless Mrs. Claus was in sight!"

I took my notepad out of my shirt and began writing this down. I knew that telling each Reindeer's story had to be the beginning of my book.

I then noticed a picture of another very young Reindeer. *Hmmm*—the antlers were almost the right size, but this Reindeer was minus the "chin whiskers." My eyes widened and I exclaimed, "Is it—could it be—Grandfather Blitzen?"

Santa threw back his head and laughed. "That's him all right, just after he won his first 'Holly Cluster' for bravery and courage. Would have been around 893. While we're having breakfast, why don't I tell the story of how Blitzen came to be lead Reindeer?"

"That would be wonderful!" I responded. "Then I'll be sure I have the details first hand."

Just then, Vixen and Prancer burst in from the kitchen and announced that breakfast was served in the dining room. While Santa and I had been talking, the other Christmas Reindeer had arrived and were seated in front of the fireplace, showing off their Christmas gifts.

I saw Donder and Dasher suddenly move to Grandfather Blitzen's side and start to help him up. He waved them away and got to his feet unassisted, grumbling, "You'd think I was 3,000 years old the way they treat me! Young scamps!" But there was a twinkle in his eye.

"They mean well, Meesha, old friend," whispered Santa, leaning down to the old Reindeer.

Puzzled, I looked at Donder and Dasher, after hearing the strange name that Santa had called Blitzen. Dasher leaned close to my ear and said, "It's his given, Christian name. Only Santa has ever used it. It means 'Forever Wisdom and Strength.'"

I glanced over at the table. Tall white and red candles lit the centerpiece of evergreen branches and holly berries. A fine linen tablecloth edged in red, green, and gold covered the table; and beautiful bone china settings were set in front of each Reindeer's assigned place.

After all heads were bowed, Santa prayed, "Almighty Father, Maker of all things, bless this table and those seated here today. Through your kindness and love we have once again completed our mission—our Christmas Eve flight. We feel your presence always, as we journey the world. Allow us to continue your chosen purpose for us. Bless the children, Father, and keep them in thy care for always and forever. And we ask this in Jesus' name. Amen."

The festive meal was hot and delicious, and the happy chatter around the table included many toasts to Christmas. The last toast was to Mrs. Claus, "For a wonderful Christmas breakfast... and just for being you!"

As we settled back into our chairs comfortably, Santa said, "And now, I promised Lad here that I would tell a remarkable story—one that you, Blitzen, will probably not care to hear again. But tell it I will. It is the story of our first-chosen Christmas Reindeer." There was great applause.

Blitzen lowered his head humbly, and Santa waited for everyone to be given a refill of hot punch before he began.

"The year was—you might have to help me, Dear," he turned to his wife.

"It was the Year of our Lord 321, Dear," she said.

Santa nodded, smiling, and continued. "Ah, yes, 321. I had been delivering toys for many years. Mrs. Claus and I would work all year alone, carving and painting each toy. Of course, in those days my journey was not quite as long as it is today. And I had a much smaller sleigh—a sled, really. However, my journey would take me through many villages, and usually through heavy snows.

"I was always very tired by the time I returned home. Christmas magic was growing, but it wasn't what it is today. Yet Mrs. Claus and I could always feel stirrings of the magic each time we loaded the sleigh on Christmas Eve.

"The problem was, the list of children's wishes kept growing longer; I couldn't keep up with the demand, one man alone making all those deliveries, pulling a sled loaded with toys behind me, as I walked on foot. That year, I didn't think I could even make it to the first village.

"Yet something about the great star, and the love I felt all about me, made me realize that that would be a very special Christmas Eve. As I set out on my journey, I looked back at Mrs. Claus waving me Godspeed, and her voice came drifting over the snow, "You must hurry, Nicholas, for tonight is very special."

"It was when I was in the small village of Geldrop, in the southern Netherlands, that I felt that warm feeling returning, making me shiver with love. Geldrop is really no different from so many small places I had visited making my deliveries—a simple village of woodcutters and farmers. Good, honest people. The children's stockings were as full as they should be, hanging from the mantelpieces. There were even snacks set out for me in those days.

"As I knelt in the snow outside the small village church, I heard a voice. It seemed more like the sound of a gentle wind—yet it was calling to me. 'Who is it? Who knows my name?' I asked.

"The voice whispered, *'Don't be afraid, Nicholas.* I have been sent to you by the Ancient of Ancients. The burden you bear grows heavier, your journey longer each year. The love of all children surrounds you and protects you as you travel.'

"'Who is speaking to me?' I queried.

"'You know me, Nicholas. I am the hopes and dreams of all children. I am the innocence of eternal childhood. Tonight, this very night, the Christmas Ancients have chosen one above all creatures on this earth to travel with you throughout time. It has been written in the Great Ledger of Deeds. This one will be devoted to you and will take upon himself the heavy burden you now pull by yourself. He is to be the first of many—eight in all—no more, no less. Welcome him. Guide him and love him, O Santa Claus! He is sent to travel with you upon the everlasting winds of Christmas-time, now and forever.'"

Santa wiped his eyes and said, "As the voice faded, I heard another voice. It was soft, yet pulled at my heart, guiding me. I walked to the side of the church. There, in a snowdrift in front of me, lay a small baby Reindeer. As it bleated, it looked up at me with the biggest, softest, most curious eyes. It was trying to get to its feet, but kept falling back into the snow, crying."

All of the Reindeer except Blitzen were now leaning forward, spellbound by Santa's story.

"I reached down and picked him up, cradled him in my arms, and he let me do so. He stared up at me with his big, soft, brown eyes and laid his head against my greatcoat. As I asked him where he was from, and why he was lying in such cold snow so late at night—he understood my words! I saw a silver chain with a medallion hanging from his neck, and as a single beam from the great star shone very brightly on it, I could read the words: *Meesha—Forever Wisdom and Strength*.

"I knew then, in my heart, that this little Reindeer with curious eyes would be with me forever. I bundled him in a warm blanket and placed him atop the sled. I would stop from time to time and offer him food or water, which he eagerly accepted. By the time we had made our last delivery and were headed for home, little Meesha was walking beside me.

"He was such a small thing that when he slipped under my hand that held the ropes to the sled, as if to pull it himself, I would pick him up and place him gently to one side. Finally I decided to let him see for himself that he was too small to pull the heavy sled. I slipped the rope over his shoulders and walked on ahead of him without looking back. As I turned to go back and get him, I almost stumbled over him and the sled too. This small Reindeer who had not even grown antlers yet had pulled the sled to me! There, in the snow and wind, little Meesha became the first-chosen Christmas Reindeer.

"We could never have imagined all of the many Christmas journeys and adventures that lay ahead of us, could we, old friend?" Santa leaned over and put his hand on Grandfather Blitzen's hoof. Blitzen still had his head lowered, and he mumbled something that made Santa smile.

"He thinks it is unnecessary, to bring this up—but

he knows that once I get going, there's no stopping me."

Santa took a sip of his punch, and deftly slipped a piece of chocolate over to Grandfather Blitzen.

"Mrs. Claus at once took little Meesha under her wing. With her care, he grew faster and stronger. He possessed a great curiosity, and would run around exploring everything, becoming familiar with every niche of our North Pole home quite quickly. More than once, Mrs. Claus would have to run him out of the house after he had overturned something!

"Once, after chasing him out of the kitchen with a broom, Mrs. Claus proclaimed that his Christmas name would be 'Blitzen,' which means 'Overwhelming.' And so, although he still carried his christening name of Meesha, he would be known to millions around the world as Blitzen. A fitting name for such a curious, headstrong Reindeer!

"As Christmas Eve drew ever closer, the first Christmas Eve Meesha had spent with us, he became quite restless, watching as the old sled was loaded with toys. He would take the ropes and, slipping them over his head, pull the sled around the compound through the snow... over small hills and back again. Never would a toy, or the enormous bag that held them, slip off the sled.'

Santa chuckled and smiled. "Mrs. Claus and I would watch him through the window for hours on end. And he never seemed to tire, even when more presents were added to the load.

"On Christmas Eve night, he stood outside in the cold wind, pawing the snow as if wanting to be off. He would run to us and slip the ropes over his head and shoulders to show us, and then stamp the ground some more. I had made my decision weeks earlier that little Meesha would have his chance. He would pull the Christmas sled and accompany me on my deliveries.

"Mrs. Claus and I slipped that first harness around his shoulders, and hooked him into the old sled. At that moment, he was the happiest Reindeer in the world!

"As I waved good-bye to Mrs. Claus, the little Reindeer that I had found in the snow one year earlier fell in behind me, his now fully grown antlers gleaming in the moonlight.

"And so, Meesha became the first Christmas Reindeer that Christmas Eve. In all the years following, he considered pulling *an even larger, new sleigh* that we had built to be his unique responsibility. *Yet his first love became the children of the world.* They were the ones he pulled the sleigh for. And he has never let them down, for all of these centuries. For many years, he pulled the sleigh alone. Yet the list continued to grow, and after almost 200 years we both knew that there was no way we could continue to do it all.

"And so, in the year 506, after our Christmas Eve journey, I confronted Meesha with our problem. He too had seen it coming. We had to figure out a way to reach all the children or Christmas deliveries would cease to exist.

"'I will find a way,' Meesha assured me. 'Aye, I will find a way!'

"I continued toy production simply on what Meesha had told me. He would find a way to cover the land in a single night. There were long periods of time during which neither I nor Mrs. Claus would see Meesha. I never questioned Meesha when he did show up after many days. He would return weary with exhaustion, only to be gone the next morning when we arose."

Santa looked up thoughtfully and whispered, "I discovered one day where he had been during his long absence. I had gone for a walk, and I sat down on a hill overlooking the ice flats, trying to think what I was going to do as Christmas was nearly upon us. I could see a small speck moving very fast across the clear ice. It was Meesha! Never had I seen such speed! Meesha blistered across the ice flats. A long trail of blue flames shot out from behind him and sparkled and glittered like thousands of prisms reflecting the sunlight. The laughter of thousands of children reached my ears as Meesha waltzed on the wind-currents of Christmas magic!"

Santa took a deep breath. "When Meesha landed, I heard the voices of the Christmas Ancients, as a sense of timelessness held me in its grasp: *Meesha, first-chosen of the Christmas Reindeer, your persistence and devoted love of all children has been rewarded. We are the care-givers and protectors of all the Christmas Reindeer. Eight in all, no more, no less! Upon you has been bestowed a great and wonderful gift. The gift of flight! Use it wisely, Meesha, and forever you shall be able to navigate the eternal songs of the winds and hold the secrets of the stars!*

"And thus was our Meesha given the gift which he now shares with the other seven Reindeer: the ability to fly, pulling my sleigh to the ends of the earth. He had found a way to reach all the children of the world. Now, on Christmas Eve, we flew over the land—and the laughter of the children was within Meesha forever. To watch as he climbed the stair steps of icy wind-currents on a thousand breezes filled my heart

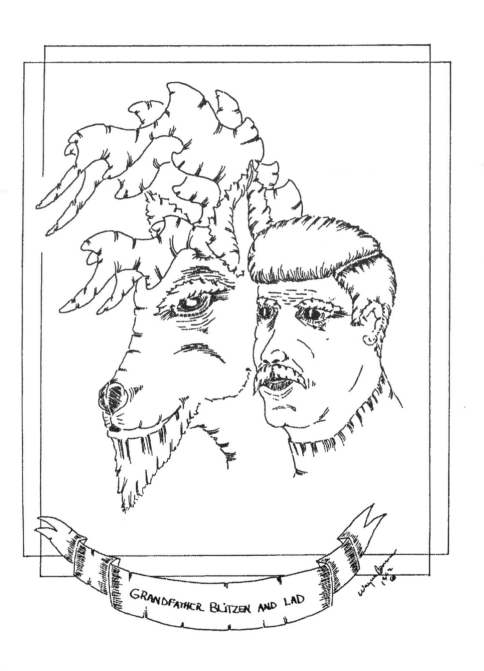

with pride for Meesha, the first-chosen Reindeer!"

Cupid was gripping my hand with excitement as she listened to Santa's story. Tears ran freely down her face, as they did on all the Christmas Reindeer. Cupid whispered, "Oh, Grandfather, how I love you…"

Santa continued: "And that is how Blitzen became the first-chosen Christmas Reindeer, and how he captured the secrets of the stars. He has remained loyal to the children of the world for nearly 1,700 mortal years. He trained each one of you, and although he grumbles sometimes when you make a mistake, you all know how very much he loves you. You are his world, his children."

When the story was over, Santa stood up and started to clap his hands. Each Reindeer stood, as I did, tears streaming down our faces as we also applauded the majestic old Reindeer. The trembling of his strong shoulders told us all that he was softly crying. Mrs. Claus went around the table and hugged him tightly and whispered ever so softly, "I'm so very proud of you, my curious little Meesha."

Santa motioned for us to follow him into the living room. We all left with Mrs. Claus still holding the old Reindeer tightly around his shoulders, both of them swaying to each other's tears of happiness and love.

11

A Visit with Santa and a Ride with Comet

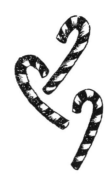

We stayed at Santa's house for about two more hours, talking and sharing stories about Christmases past. I told them how I had waited up one Christmas Eve when I was about ten, so that I could talk with them. Santa, stroking his beard, interrupted by saying, "I remember that, don't you, Donder?"

"Yes," said Donder, "didn't we find him asleep in front of the fireplace with a letter clutched in his hand, telling us to wake him up when we got there?"

Santa laughed heartily, "That's right, Lad. We walked all around you and made quite a bit of noise, but you never opened your eyes. And it's against our rules to wake any child, except in an emergency."

Sadly, I said, "I was really disappointed. Mom and Dad had taken me to the department store to see you, but I knew it wasn't really you."

Santa smiled thoughtfully. "It couldn't have been about that bully at your school who kept stealing your lunch, could it?"

Startled, I asked, "How did you know?"

Donder spoke up. "Didn't you find a letter in your hand when you woke up the next morning? You were so excited about all of your presents that you dropped it behind the Christmas tree and forgot all about it. Your father found it and read it to you a couple of days later. It said, 'Be a good boy and trust in your dad. He'll know what to do.'"

"Yes—I remember now. Dad talked to me about how to handle the bully, and then he read the letter he said you had left for me. Did you leave it?"

"Did *you* leave it, Donder?" Santa asked the Reindeer.

Donder grinned. "Sure. I was worried about you. Every boy needs to eat lunch. I knew your dad would give you the right advice. I understand the bully didn't steal your lunch after that."

"He sure didn't!" I exploded. "It cost me a black eye, but I got to eat lunch every day. You were right to tell me to talk to my dad. He taught me how to stand up for myself."

After that discussion, Santa called everyone's attention to the center of the room. Santa was standing beside Dancer. "Lad, Dancer wanted me to give you this present, from him. He said that you might be afraid to open it if he tried to give it to you. And he really wants you to have it." I thought of the ugly hat with flaps that I had hurriedly stuffed into the pocket of my coat when we'd arrived.

This was a large package wrapped in shiny silver. I reached for it cautiously—surely if Santa was presenting it to me it couldn't be a trap.

The lid of the box fell as I opened it quickly. Then I held up the most beautiful red sweater. On it were woven pictures of all the Christmas Reindeer in flight, pulling the great sleigh and Santa too! Dancer had knitted the sweater himself.

I must have been beaming when I looked up. "*You*

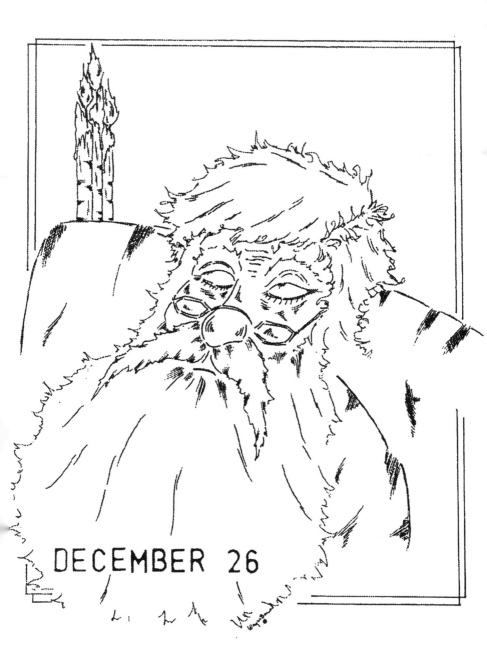

can wear it with the HAT!" Dancer whispered to me mischievously.

Then he held out his foreleg to me. "Friends?" he said.

"Of course," I answered. "I'm just sorry I didn't have anything to give you."

"Oh, but you did," interrupted Dasher. "Dancer was wearing the cutest snowball this morning when he opened his front door!"

Everyone, including Dancer, burst into laughter.

After some more friendly banter, we all realized how tired we were and started to take our leave. Donder and I were the last to go. As we put on our coats, Santa told me that each Reindeer would sleep for a day or two to recover from the strain of the past day and a half. A long afternoon nap sounded good to me too!

But they wanted me to come back tomorrow to hear Mrs. Claus tell the story of how little Cupid had become a Christmas Reindeer.

When Donder and I were alone at his house again, I exclaimed, "Without a doubt, this has been the best Christmas of my whole life!"

"But it's not over yet, Lad," Donder replied sleepily. "In a couple of days, we start again, working for Christmas next year. Santa will give each of us our work assignments—and don't be surprised if he gives you some too!"

"But—what could *I* do?" I stammered.

"You'll just have to wait and see like the rest of us."

After that, we both slept peacefully. In fact, to my surprise, I found I didn't wake up until the next morning.

A Visit with Santa and a Ride with Comet 113

I stumbled out of bed, walked over to the desk in my room, and found a note which read: "You will probably want to go exploring when you wake up. Hot chocolate and bread for toast are in the kitchen. If the clock on the wall, North Pole time, reads between 6:00 and 10:00 A.M., you can wander about freely. Everyone, including Santa, should be up. A word of caution: Stay away from the elves for now. They always sleep late for a day or two after Christmas. I should be up soon. Have fun. Donder."

After eating breakfast and bundling up in my new topcoat, I started down the hill. It was snowing and our tracks from yesterday had all been covered.

As I reached the square, I saw Comet walking toward me. "Well, you're up early!" he said, his breath making small frost clouds as he spoke.

"I was just going to explore the grounds a little..."

Comet grinned and said, "When I first arrived, I couldn't get enough of it all either. Everyone is still asleep except for Santa and you and I. I'd still be in bed too, but Santa summoned me to run an errand this morning. I have to go to Greenland, just off the coast of the Lincoln Sea, to pick up some blue ice for Mrs. Claus. She's going to make snow-cream later today and she'll only use blue ice. Hey, wanta come with me? I could sure use the company."

"Wow! That would be great!" I stammered. "Do we need to hook up the sleigh?"

"Naw, we've all got special passenger saddles that Santa had made up for us a couple of hundred years ago. You can use mine. Come on."

He turned and led the way toward the shed that held the great sleigh. Inside I saw a row of shiny saddles, one to fit each Reindeer's size. Comet put his on and I climbed aboard. He reached down and hooked a shiny bucket to collect the blue ice in.

Comet then turned to me and instructed, "Just say, 'Away, Comet, AWAY!!!!!'"

Soon we were airborne. The trees below us seemed just a blur, and I couldn't see anything of the snow but a fast-moving screen of white. It was a very smooth ride. I felt no bumps or jars at all, as I held on tightly to his antlers.

Just ahead, the coast of the Arctic Circle was racing toward us. Soon I saw the water rush by beneath us. Comet was leaving a great stardust trail behind us. Seeming satisfied, he dove to the right and stayed on a straight course for the coast of Greenland. I relaxed with my thoughts.

It almost seemed as though this speedy Reindeer were "running" through the air. He placed his front hooves out ahead of him and "dug in" with his back feet, almost as a rabbit would run through the snow. His rhythm was flawless, and he kept up a steady pace. His breath came in short spurts of cold, foggy air as he breathed. *"There it is! We're coming to it now!"* he shouted.

I saw land ahead of us, and Comet began his descent. We landed atop a small hill overlooking an enormous patch of ice. It sparkled blue, even against the falling snow. Hopping off and unhooking the bucket, I walked with him to the water's edge. He seemed to be looking for a good vein of blue ice. At a short ice wall, he began to hammer with his antlers. Chunks of ice and frozen particles flew through the air. Comet dug about two feet into the mound and uncovered the brightest blue ice I had ever seen.

"That should do us," he said, as he finished collecting the blue ice. "Ready to head back?"

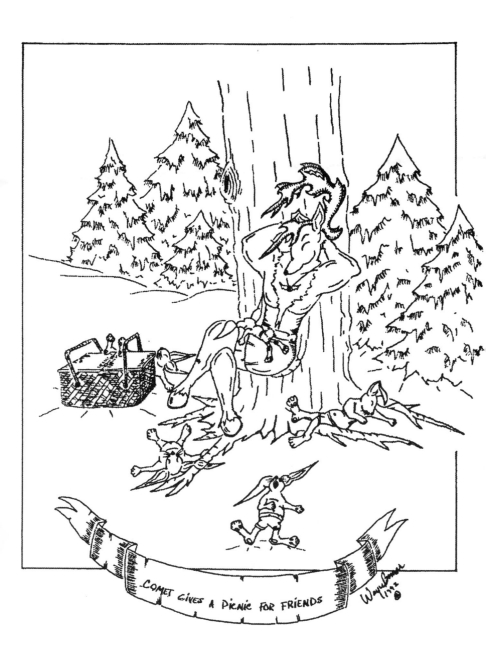

Greatly impressed, I nodded, and again climbed aboard this amazing Christmas Reindeer.

After we saw the water of the Arctic Ocean rushing under us, and I guess we were about halfway back home, he yelled: "Hang on tight! I want to try some sharp maneuvers I've been practicing!!"

Crouching low to his back, I wrapped my fingers around the girth strap and squeezed my knees against Comet's flanks. Feeling that I was secure, Comet started driving even harder and faster with his back legs. With a sudden movement of his front feet, I felt myself going end over end in a dizzying, whirling motion.

As my stomach started to turn over (I had had three cups of hot chocolate that morning!) I felt us climbing high—and then we dove. Comet stretched his front legs along his side flanks and took up a falcon-like dive. Opening my eyes a little, I could see the water boiling toward us at an unbelievable speed.

Just when I thought we would plunge into the turbulent sea, Comet banked very sharply to the left, which left me hanging in thin air. Comet surged instantly under me, laughing loudly, and I scrambled upright onto his back. I again took my clamped-knee position and he started to climb even higher!

Higher, higher, we went—until I thought we might need the star mask. Then, pausing a moment, he dove for the coast of the North Pole.

A mile or so inland, he again leveled out and softly hit the frozen snow running. Inside of five minutes, we were back at the shed. As I helped Comet put the saddle back in its place, I couldn't stop praising him about his speed and graceful maneuvers.

What a great addition my ride with Comet would be to my book about the Christmas Reindeer!

We took the blue ice to Mrs. Claus, and she gave us cups of hot chocolate to warm us up after our run. Glancing out her kitchen window, she said, "Well, here comes Santa. I had better start the snow cream now. You will join us, won't you two? After all, I couldn't be making it if you hadn't gone to get the blue ice."

Comet and I both nodded.

"Good. We'll see you around 4:00, North Pole time. Comet, why don't you take Lad down to the Toy Factory and show him around until then."

As we were heading that way, Donder came and caught up with us. "Mind if I join you?"

Soon we came to an enormous building from which we could hear a great deal of noise coming. Comet held the door open for us and we all stepped inside. The place was alive with elves! It scared me a little, they were rushing about so. They even ran into each other, knocking themselves down and just getting up as though nothing had happened.

"They're just waking up!" shouted Donder. "Don't get in their way. They have to get their heads on straight before they can calm down."

It was so hectic inside the Toy Factory that Day After Christmas that we ended up bolting out the back door. "Whew, that was close!" said Donder.

"Do they always act like that when they're working?" I asked.

"Oh, they're not working now. We call it 'elf swarming,' and unless you like that sort of melee, I suggest you avoid them for a few days. Then they'll get settled down some. But, actually, Christmas wouldn't be Christmas without them. They do most of the work, you know—and more than just making toys. They have many skills."

Donder started laughing. "Grandfather Blitzen calls them eager little 'snippers,' the way they always fuss over him. He says that when you stare at an elf, it will bring you good luck, right, Comet?"

"That's right."

We were all looking for something to do next—an adventure that would teach me about the North Pole so that I could write about it in my book.

"I know," said Donder, "let's go wake up Vixen and take a walk with her over to the Valley of Christmas Trees. I bet Lad would really enjoy seeing that."

Comet nodded, and we turned up the hill that led to the Reindeer compound. Just ahead of us was Vixen's house. I thought of the many questions I had for her.

We had come to the next walkway which led to Vixen's front door. Beautiful red poinsettias lined her shoveled walk.

Excitedly, we approached her door. I was dying for a look at a whole valley of Christmas Trees and the story they would reveal to me!

12

A Visit with Vixen and the Valley of Christmas Trees

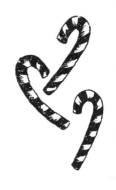

Donder knocked very gently on Vixen's door. We heard the sound of footsteps... and then the door opened. Vixen smiled at us. "Come in, come in!"

As Comet, Donder, and I entered, she waved us to her living room. "Sit down. Make yourselves comfortable. I'll get us something to drink."

Glancing around her living room showed me that Vixen was a Reindeer with fine, neat taste. Her Christmas tree was exquisite—it was decorated with tiny crystal ornaments of all sizes and shapes. And the candles that lit her tree reflected shimmering beams of light on the crystal decorations.

Just to the side of her fireplace was a reading and writing desk. Apparently she had been writing just before we came. There were pictures of children on it—and in other places around the room. Her medals and awards were hung inside a glass frame just over the fireplace. A small chandelier hung from the center of the room—all lit in green candles.

Her front, bay window had a bench seat, and I somehow felt that Vixen probably sat looking out of that window for hours at a time.

Just then she came back into the room with a tray. On it were four mugs of hot, steaming punch. "I thought everyone might be getting tired of hot chocolate!" she said, smiling. "I hope you like it. It's my own recipe."

"Excellent!" I responded, delighted with the smell of cinnamon and hint of nutmeg that always made me think of holidays.

"I'm really glad you came over," she said. "I was just writing thank-you notes to the children, and I really got stumped while writing one. It is to a little girl named Ellen. You remember her, Donder. She's the one who never fails to leave us candy canes in stockings that she crochets herself."

Donder nodded. "Yes, I remember Ellen. Isn't she still in the hospital?"

"Yes," answered Vixen sadly. "She still didn't forget us, though. Remember she had her father leave the candy canes outside for us this year?"

"That's right. How is she now? Is she getting any better?"

Vixen lowered her head and said, "I don't know if we will find those candy canes from her next year. She's slipping away from us…"

Vixen turned sideways in her chair and said, "I'm not sure if I should ask you, Lad—but do you think you could help me find the right words to put down? I just can't seem to gather my thoughts clearly—when I think of how sick she is, and how uncertain she is of even seeing another Christmas!"

"I'm honored that you want my help. I'll certainly try my best to help you write something that will cheer her up."

Donder and Comet stood up, draining their mugs

down. Comet said, "Why don't we come back for you two later? We'll walk up to Christmas Tree Valley. Maybe by then, everyone else will be up."

"Hey, Vixen," Donder added. "Don't be too hard on yourself. We do what we can, and then we must leave the rest to the Father. Ellen's in good hands, either way."

We said good-bye to the other two.

"Ellen's just so special to me," Vixen confided after they had gone out. *"She truly believes in us.* So strongly, I can feel it. Donder's always warning me not to get too personally involved with the children, but sometimes it's hard not to. There are so many with problems. I wish I could help them all! But I feel as though I do go deeper into these people's lives than the other Reindeer do—except perhaps for Blitzen."

"Vixen, I think it's wonderful that you try to help. Sometimes I hurt so much for someone else that I can hardly stand it. I like to feel, if enough people will wish strongly enough, that, like a prayer, our thoughts will help and even *heal.* Ellen believes in you and you know it. What better gift can one give than the gift of love?"

Vixen was cheered.

"Now," I smiled. "Vixen, let me tell you a story about a little boy. Many years ago, this boy looked forward to Christmas. Every year, he would eagerly await Santa and his magical Reindeer. He was never forgotten; he even kept the letters that the Reindeer left for him. He felt immense joy at having something that had come from these special Reindeer—just to him.

"Sometimes he would go to school, or on picnics, or play baseball, or do all the other ordinary things that little boys do. But he never forgot the magical Reindeer.

"However, in time, he grew up. Other people made fun of him because he still believed in the Reindeer and the magic of Christmas. They would laugh at him and tell him to grow up and stop being a child.

"The boy—who by now was a grown man—was very unhappy because he felt the world was pushing him into giving up believing. He continued to work and do all the things that grownup men do; but every Christmas Eve he would feel depressed because the magical Reindeer of Christmas would not stop at his house again.

"He stopped leaving food for them, and on Christmas morning there would be no letter to cheer him. Christmas for him was fading. The years passed, and the man saw many changes in how people celebrated Christmas. It didn't seem to mean the same things that it had during his childhood.

"Then, one Christmas, the young man went to church. He didn't know why—maybe for the company of other people. As he sat and listened to the sermon—which was the Christmas story—he felt inside that *the magic wasn't gone. He* had been the one who had shut it out. He had forgotten all of the joy that comes with Christmas.

"After church, the young man went home, and for whatever reason he couldn't explain—maybe a warm feeling, maybe love—the man once again left food for the magical Reindeer and Santa Claus. He also left a short letter reading: 'I have missed you terribly. Can you forgive me? With Love...'

"The next morning, the young man woke and, rushing to the door, threw it open. There on the ground beside the empty plate was a small gift and a letter!

"Tearing open the letter, he read: 'We have missed you also. Can you forgive *us*? Signed, All of Us, with Love.'

"The young man found his magic again. The joy he felt when he found the letter and the gift brought the magic flooding back. He cried tears of happiness —someone cared about him! They had asked for *his* forgiveness.

"This young man still carries the magic of Christmas and the magical Reindeer in his heart. People might laugh and make fun of him, but what does that matter? He truly believes, and that's all that's important."

Through all of this story, Vixen was listening attentively. When I was finished, she drew an old envelope out of her desk drawer—one that had yellowed with age. She handed it to me. I read it once again: *"I have missed you terribly. Can you forgive me? With Love..."*

"We never doubted your belief," she said. "We just felt that maybe somewhere along the line, growing up, you had got sidetracked. We always passed over your house and looked for your letters. It was Grandfather Blitzen who kept telling us, when he would see our disappointed faces, that one day we would find letters from you waiting for us again.

"'That one will never lose the magic,' he'd say. And sure enough, one Christmas Eve, your letter was there. Grandfather Blitzen wrote the reply, and I wrapped the small gift. It was something special that we keep on hand for those who find the magic again."

I slowly pulled out the small silver chain from around my neck and read the medallion that said, *"Merry Christmas... Again."*

"Yes! The magic is still alive," I affirmed, fingering the medallion. "And not just on Christmas Eve, but throughout the year. It took me a long time to realize that."

"And that's why you're finally here," said Vixen. Then, turning her thoughts to the small child who was ill, she said, "Thank you. I can write to Ellen now, and I know I'll have the exact words to say. You've helped me more than you know."

I sat beside Vixen as she wrote. She never faltered, though she wrote quickly. Finishing, she sealed it in an envelope and pressed the Christmas Reindeer seal of hot wax against the flap. Walking across the room, she put the envelope in a clear tube that ran up her wall in the corner. The letter disappeared with a soft *whooshing* sound. "The elves will see that it's mailed," she said.

Vixen sat back down and for a while we talked further of what Christmas meant to both of us. Suddenly, she grinned and said, "Let's go find Donder and Comet and take that walk up to Christmas Tree Valley. I feel so much better, and I really want you to see the trees."

As Vixen put on her topcoat and opened the door, she turned and said, "Thanks for everything."

"Anytime," I returned.

We had just started down her front steps when Donder and Comet bounded up. "Where are you headed?" asked Donder?

"We were just going up to Christmas Tree Valley. I want to show him that marvel," explained Vixen.

Comet led the way. Our path was completely covered with fresh snow. I tried to step in Donder's tracks, as the deep snow made tough walking for ahuman. I was constantly amazed at the natural wonders of the North Pole.

The falling snow glistened like a shower of diamonds, and the wind seemed to play melodies. We walked slowly. The Reindeer seemed to know that I wanted to see everything. A short time later, we stopped on a hill overlooking a spectacular sight.

There in front of us, in a little valley, were hundreds of evergreen trees, all decorated for Christmas. Through the falling snow, the sparkling lights blazed forth, and each tree was the colors of a thousand rainbows.

The winding path took us through the maze of lights and sparkles. Each tree was labeled with a metal plaque just in front of it. There were trees from each country of the world, decorated as they would have been in that country. There were trees from America, Russia, Brazil, Australia, Denmark, the Netherlands, Canada... the list went on and on.

Although the snow fell and the wind blew, each tree stood fast and did not waver. Not one decoration fell to the ground. It was perfectly still in the little valley.

I ran here and there among the trees and for long minutes felt lost in a sea of Christmas.

Donder, Comet, and Vixen must have had a hard time keeping up with me. They ran behind me if they thought I might have missed one. Then they would point it out. I had never in all my dreams imagined all of this existed.

Vixen pointed to a small house on the outskirts of the valley. "Just there, lives the tree keeper. An old elf named Wick. He's been doing it for centuries. Keeps up with all the latest fashions and trends for Christmas trees."

Donder remarked, "He keeps very much to himself—might come down to the Great Hall every now and then, and we always leave something in his stocking. Other than that, we rarely see him."

"Cupid's in pretty good with old Wick. You might ask her about him. She comes down here quite often to see if he's all right or needs anything. Wick even did a special tree for her. Come on, we'll show you," said Comet.

Eagerly, walking fast behind them, I followed them to a small clearing just off the path.

"There it is," said Vixen. The metal plaque in front of the small evergreen read "Cupid's Tree." Her tree was about fifteen feet high, and it was decorated with small symbols of Cupid in all colors. Each decoration looked like blown glass, and each little detail was outstanding. The little tree was a fitting symbol of its namesake—expressing how much Cupid loved everyone.

Walking back the way we had come, I turned once more so that I might keep in my mind the beautiful Christmas Tree Valley, the work of the elf Wick. Silently we turned and headed for the Reindeer compound.

Donder suddenly stopped in his tracks and sniffed the air. "Snow cream!" he shouted enthusiastically. It was almost 4:00 P.M., and Comet and I looked at each other, thinking about our invitation to the Clauses' house. I didn't know if we should bring Vixen and Donder as well.

Comet edged closer to me. "It's all right," he assured me. "She'll be expecting us and several others to share the snow cream."

Feeling better about us all descending on the

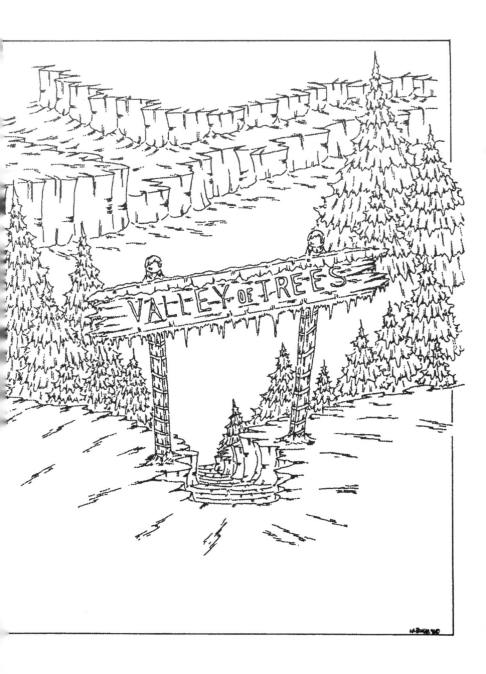

Clauses, I was delighted when we arrived at their back door. I could hear Santa and Mrs. Claus laughing, and then Santa's voice, "You know, Dear, when you make this stuff, sooner or later, all of the Reindeer are going to be knocking on our door!"

When we knocked, they smiled and welcomed us in. After we had enjoyed the marvelous treat, they invited us into the living room by the fireplace.

"What a day," Santa said, yawning. "I hope all of the elves are fully awake in a day or so. We have to get busy for next year. By the way, Dear," he said, turning to his wife. "Now would be a good time to tell the story of little Cupid and how she came to be with us. You're definitely the one to tell it."

"Very well." Mrs. Claus smiled. "It's so cozy here by the fire that I do feel like chatting."

I got out my notepad and wrote "Cupid" at the top of the page, as Mrs. Claus began to tell the story of the youngest and smallest Christmas Reindeer. I was all ears.

13

The Littlest Christmas Reindeer

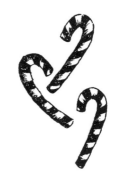

For a moment, Mrs. Claus stared into the crackling fire, gathering her thoughts. She quickly wiped her eyes, and, turning to us, said, "Her name is Elsker, which means 'Love with Fond Devotion.' It was the year 1269. I remember it quite well. Our other children—that is, the Reindeer—had grown so, and it was a very happy time. There was lots of bustling about...

"The list of toys was ever so much longer by then. The making and packing and delivering had turned into a full-time job for all of us.

"For once, the world seemed to be in a state of calm. The spirit of Christmas that year was overwhelming. But to me, there was something lacking. I didn't know what it was!

"Everyone was quite organized, and our plans seemed to be going so well—just three days before Christmas Eve. All of the children were being refitted for their new starshoes; and the elves—oh, my, you could hear them singing all the way up here from the Great Hall of Toys!

"Santa was in fine spirits. Yet still I felt there was more. It was almost like the feeling I had in 320, when Blitzen had joined us. It had been so long since I'd felt like that. I was Blitzen who came to me shortly before the Christmas Eve journey began that year. I had never seen him quite look or act as he was doing. He told me he felt a hurting—not within himself, but of something that seemed to call him from far away.

"He himself had worried long about this matter. He had awakened at night from sleep, night after night, for months. He sensed an extreme loneliness—yet it was nothing he could actually put his hoof on. I told him I sensed something like that too.

"The more we talked about it, the better we began to feel. It was as though this terrible loneliness and fear were going to end soon. He turned to go, and just before he walked outside, he said, 'Tonight, we will go to Lapland first. I feel...'

"He said no more, but I saw him out by the sleigh conferring with Santa. They were giving new directions for Dancer to navigate the path, to reroute toward Lapland. As they took off, Blitzen had turned to me in the doorway where I stood and smiled specially. I knew in my heart that he would fix whatever had been wrong.

"Wishing them Godspeed, my heart lifted. And now I will tell you what Blitzen did—as he related it to me after their return.

"I was wondering when they would get back, it seemed like a longer trip than usual. Then I heard the bells and finally a soft knock on the door. When I opened it, there stood Blitzen in the soft, falling snow. In his arms was the smallest, frailest reindeer I had ever seen!

"Blitzen had the biggest smile on his face. He extended his forelegs to me and I took the little reindeer from him. He said, 'This tiny thing was the cause of our worry. Her name is Elsker.'

"I held the little reindeer, whose tiny heart was pounding so hard it frightened me. She looked around, very scared, and it was only when Blitzen took her again that she seemed to calm down. He sat by the fireplace for a while and cuddled her, singing softly to her. I prepared a toy doll bottle with warm milk for her, and went to get some blankets. As Blitzen wrapped the little thing in the blankets and fed her, he told me her story.

"'As we neared the Arctic Circle, my feelings had become stronger—I was sure someone was calling to me. I led the team faster, following my inner instinct. We had just started across the Lofoten Islands in the Norwegian Sea. My feelings were so strong that I descended, quite to everyone's surprise. I circled a small island in the group of which I think had no name—landing on the ice and slipping my traces.

"'I could hear Santa Claus calling to me as I ran. My loyalty to him sent me back to the team, in spite of how I felt. They must have thought me crazy. Then, as I turned back, I heard little Elsker whimper. There, beneath a half-buried log, I found her, crying and starving. As I picked her up, I cried, seeing the condition she was in. I sat in the cold snow and held her, my tears falling on her.'"

Mrs. Claus stopped her story for a minute and looked at us. "Blitzen never told anyone but me of his feelings that night. I now have his permission to share them with you."

Donder, Comet, and Vixen nodded, their faces aglow.

Mrs. Claus continued. "Blitzen told me how he gathered up the little reindeer and brought her back to the sleigh. He laid her beside Santa, and they continued on, of course. But only after Blitzen had seen to her need for warmth, and she had eaten something.

"My good Santa kept one hand on her the entire flight, to comfort her. Each Reindeer slipped his traces at each stop and offered what he or she could to the weak little Elsker. I was told that somewhere during the flight, the feelings of love and magic among the Reindeer so overpowered them that they had to land.

"Rushing back to the sleigh, they all saw that Santa was holding baby Elsker up and smiling. He had boomed out in his great voice that 'She'll be all right now. Food and warmth and love will cure the littlest reindeer!'

"A feeling of joy swept through all of them, and with happy hearts they renewed their journey, gathering up into flight all the magic of Christmas Eves past. It was that year that many Endurance Medals were awarded for nonstop flight!

"Little Elsker sat beside Santa and begged for Blitzen at each stop. Then, after all the deliveries had been completed, they happily headed for home. That was when Blitzen brought her to me, and I began to care for her.

"Each of you, I remember, would come by and get her from time to time. I watched you walk off with little Elsker skipping around you. I thought how loving and caring you all were. Donder would pull her for hours over the snow in the old sled. How she loved that and would squeal with laughter when Donder would fly a foot or two above the ground!

"Then, all of us began to notice things about Elsker. She could button her topcoat by herself, and she spent long minutes sitting by Santa's boots, tying and retying the long shoelaces. Quite extraordinary for such a small, young reindeer. She was truly nimble and quick—doing things with her hooves that amazed even old Blitzen.

"Blitzen came and got me one afternoon and said he had something I had to see. We went to the old shed where the great sleigh was stored. Peeping in, I saw little Elsker. She had taken down all the harnesses and had hooked them to the sleigh in perfect order. Her tiny hooves moved so fast, I had to watch quickly.

"She made no mistakes. Blitzen and I checked it later. Everything was in perfect order—every knot and hook just right and tightened just so. Santa could not have done it better himself."

Santa nodded his head as if in answer to Mrs. Claus.

"That evening as Elsker was eating her supper and Blitzen and I were alone in the living room talking, I asked him how he had taught her to handle the harnesses. He shook his great antlers and said, "Twas not I. I never even showed her where the great sleigh was stored.'

"Puzzled, we asked each of you if sometimes in your walks with her you had shown her how to hook in the heavy harness and hooks. The reply was always no.

"Elsker grew much stronger, and we watched as she displayed her deftness with complicated hitches and knots. A wonderful thought began to grow in our minds. The next Christmas Eve I watched Santa and the elves hitch up the Reindeer. Little Elsker was right there helping harness each of you for flight.

"She double-checked each hook and stitch. Seeming satisfied that nothing was loose, she came back to stand by me. As we both watched you disappear into the night sky on your journey, Elsker looked very happy. She watched until she couldn't see even a speck in the sky. And, anxiously awaiting your return, she ran outside as soon as she heard the bells announcing you were near.

"After your landing, she was there to unharness the hitches—she was half finished before the elves could get to it. They too were amazed as she did it all so neatly and swiftly. Santa and I watched as each of you congratulated her on her work, and told her how much you had missed her."

Comet then spoke up. "Yes, we missed her greatly. And so we went to you…"

"Yes," said Mrs. Claus. "But I think we had already made up our minds."

Santa smiled and nodded and reached for his pipe. "Yes," he concurred. "One afternoon, not long afterward, I sent Elsker to the toy factory to see if she could help any of the elves. It was my way of getting her out of the house while we all talked. I had no doubts, however, about the outcome. Little Elsker was to join the team!"

"Yes," continued Mrs. Claus. "She had proven her worth, and she was greatly loved as well. But at the time, not one of us said a word to Elsker about the decision. So as Christmas Eve eventually approached again, she diligently began going to the shed to check the harness and traces, even altering some to fit you more exactly. And she attached small silver bells to each harness and fitted them perfectly into the heavy tracings.

"She even made some presents for you: mittens, hoof slippers, antler coverings. And she took on extra chores so that you all could concentrate on Christmas

Eve preparations. Finally we had to tell her to slow down—she was overly anxious to 'pull her weight.' But she would only smile and ask, 'Isn't there anything else I can do?'

"Fact was, she had one desire that she never mentioned. Her dream was to become one of the Christmas Reindeer herself. She thought she was too little and weak to be included with Reindeer who had centuries of experience behind them. So she kept her dream a secret.

"The months passed, and little Elsker grew into a beautiful, graceful reindeer. Then, on Christmas Eve, the great sleigh was pulled from its place in the shed, all sparkling and clean, with runners waxed. Elsker stayed with the sleigh and watched the loading of the toys. Then the elves brought the heavy harness around, and she looked on with pride as you all got into your positions. She started forward to hitch you into the tracings, as she had done the year before.

"But Santa stopped her and asked if she would run down to the toy factory to fetch a special gift just inside the door—he said he'd almost forgotten it. She looked disappointed that she wouldn't get to hook up the Reindeer again, but she obeyed Santa without hesitation.

"When she returned, she saw that the elves had already tightened the cinches and girth straps and that you were all safely hitched in. Sadly, she handed the special gift Santa had requested to the elf who was putting last-minute orders into the sleigh. Then Elsker came to stand by me.

"The elf, who was, I believe, Mergen, said, 'Why, Elsker, this gift's for you. Santa, might she open it now?'

"Elsker, on hearing her name, turned and looked at Santa. As he nodded, she opened the package. A shiny new harness fell at her feet—it was complete with small silver bells that jingled upon hitting the ground! She stared at you all, not daring to hope.

"It was then that she noticed your positions. Why was Donder standing beside Grandfather Blitzen, when he usually stood alone out front? Why was there an empty place beside Dasher, just in front of the sleigh? He usually ran beside Prancer. *Why was everyone grinning and Santa Claus laughing so loudly?*

"'Well, we're all waiting!' Santa finally boomed, sweeping his red-robed arm toward the empty position beside Dasher.

"There were shouts of congratulations and much applauding from the elves. Little Elsker ran to stand beside Dasher. After being completely harnessed in, she stood proud and erect, shaking with nervousness, awaiting takeoff. I whispered to her how very proud we were of her, and that she would do just fine.

"I remember Blitzen's very words: "Tis complete we are now, aye! Eight in all, no more, no less! From among all reindeer, she has been chosen to fulfill immortal Christmas destiny—to bring love and cheer to all the children of the world. Behold our Cupid, for this is, now and forever, to be her Christmas name. You, Cupid, are now a Christmas Reindeer!'"

Mrs. Claus paused thoughtfully and dabbed at her eyes with a handkerchief. "As they took off into the atmosphere that night, I could just faintly hear Santa say for the first time, 'Away, my little Cupid, away!'"

I was so touched by Cupid's story that it was difficult to write parts of it down as I heard it. Mrs. Santa wisely broke the heavy emotional tone of the moment

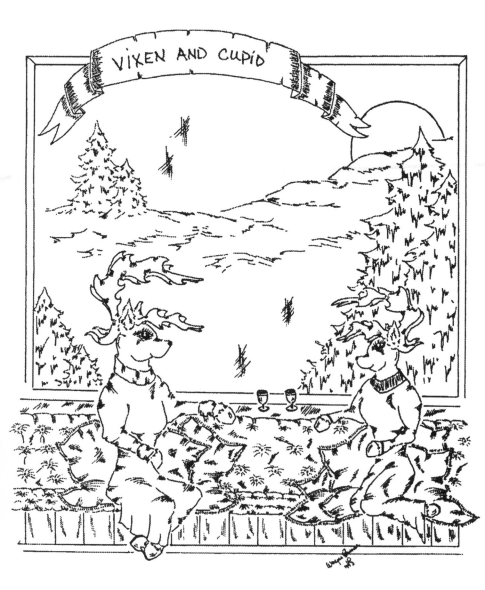

by announcing, "I think some nice, hot chocolate would be good right now!"

Vixen hurried after her to help. Comet poked me with his arm and pointed to Santa. He was sound asleep, his arms folded over his chest. We all got up quietly to go into the kitchen, so as not to wake him. When we finally left by the back door, saying our good-byes to Mrs. Claus, we concluded that it had been a perfect evening.

14

Santa's Christmas Assignments and Vixen's Workroom

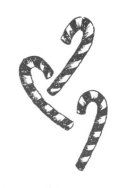

I was awakened the next morning by Donder's gentle shaking. "Come on, sleepyhead, time to get up. The hour is later than you think! We've both overslept!"

Sleepily, I looked at my friend, then realized he had been up first. The aroma from the kitchen was unmistakable! Hotcakes and tea. I hurried to the breakfast table he had prepared.

"What's happening today?" I asked, curious as to what a North Pole schedule turned into after Christmas.

"Santa is going to give Christmas assignments to everyone this morning," he answered. "We need to get over to the Great Hall of Toys as soon as possible."

After eating and cleaning up, we dashed out. Hurrying down the hill toward the Great Hall of Toys, we met up with Dasher, Comet, and Vixen, who also seemed in a hurry.

When we arrived and entered the Hall, we found it alive with confusion and chattering elves. Santa was on a stage in the center with Newton, his chief elf, and Grandfather Blitzen standing beside him. The desk in front of them held a pile of stacked-up papers. What mysteries did those papers hold? I wondered.

I was curious as to what kind of assignment Santa would give me. With Blitzen's help, Santa started handing out orders to different elves, and they hurried off to their own departments to begin preparations. It really didn't take that long for him to work through the pile of lists. Newton finally handed each order out to whomever Santa designated for the job. Pretty soon no one was left in the Hall but the Reindeer, Santa, and I.

Santa cleared his throat. "First, I want Dancer and Prancer to see to the new harness that was ordered last year. The harness department has just finished with the new rigging. You two, assisted by Cupid, will see to it that all the harnesses fit each of you perfectly. Cupid, you will check the hooks and cinches. I want you also to fit each buckle into the shoulder harnesses—and the bells must be placed just right. Any questions?"

Dancer and Prancer nodded their agreement. Cupid smiled and said, "We'll take care of it, Santa."

With that, the three of them hurried off to the back of the Hall, where the harness department was located.

Turning to us, Santa said, "Comet, you and Dasher will be in charge of production of the new line of stuffed animals that the fabric department is working on. Each stitch must be just right, each toy must be perfect. You must see to it that the legs and feet are properly formed—and make sure the elves match the tails with the right animals!"

That left Donder, Vixen, and me. Blitzen handed Santa several papers which he checked carefully, asking Blitzen some questions we couldn't hear. Then Santa looked up at Blitzen, smiling. He called Donder and me forward, clearing his throat to present us with our orders for next year's preparation.

"It seems that a most difficult assignment has been issued to both of you," he began soberly. "It's going to require a lot of responsibility—but Blitzen seems to feel you can handle it."

"Whatever you want us to do, Santa," assured Donder, "we'll do our best."

Santa smiled. "I know you will. Blitzen seems to think you make a pretty good team. He will stand by to give you the support you will need."

I was getting nervous. What did Santa expect of us—of me?

"You two will be responsible for setting up appointments with the other Christmas Reindeer and myself concerning Lad's interviewing process. You must schedule each Reindeer in such a way that it doesn't interfere with their assigned tasks. Donder, you are to guide Lad through the entire North Pole operation and explain to him how everything works here." Santa grinned at Donder. "And that includes the mailroom!" Donder let out a groan.

Santa continued, "You're not to miss a thing. You certainly know about all our routines here, as the second-lead Reindeer. You are also to make sure that Lad has sufficient writing materials. I expect a lot of this interviewing will need to be done at night, after the Reindeer have finished their work day. And get him a tape recorder!"

As Santa talked, Donder had been quickly taking notes. "Where will the interviews be conducted?" he asked finally.

"You may choose time and place, Donder. But make sure you're present if Lad interviews Dancer one-on-one. I don't want Lad to be given any wild tales about how he saved Mars or Jupiter!"

Santa pointed at me next. "And now you!"

I cringed, I guess visibly, because Santa assured me, "Never fear, Lad. What I have in mind will be most enjoyable."

I relaxed a little, and reached for the notebook Santa was handing me. "These are questions we find are most asked by children and grownups alike about the Christmas Reindeer. Do try to incorporate the answers to these questions into your stories."

"Certainly, Santa," I replied. "It will be my pleasure."

"The best of luck to you, Lad."

And with that, Santa Claus turned and walked toward the main toy assembly plant. I turned to Donder, who was talking with Blitzen.

"Tonight at 6:00, North Pole time, would be fine. I'll expect everyone," said Blitzen, who then turned and hurried after Santa and Newton.

"What was that all about?" I asked curiously.

"Oh, that is the appointment for Blitzen to tell us the story of how Vixen became a Christmas Reindeer in 921."

That rang a bell. Vixen hadn't been present at the handing out of assignments. "Where is she?" I asked. "Santa didn't give her any assignments. She'll be so hurt..."

"Don't worry about Vixen, Lad," Donder assured me. "She already has her orders—they're the same every year."

"What is her standing assignment then?"

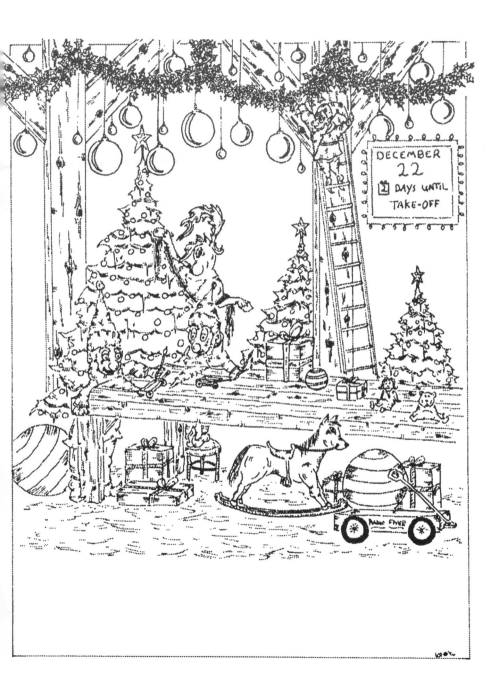

Donder grinned. "Vixen is in charge of the North Pole mailroom. And that's one job I wouldn't want for anything! She's definitely got her work cut out for her. She's the one who reads all those letters sent to us by children. This time of year, it's not too bad—but wait until the first of September!"

"You mean she's the one who decides who's 'naughty' or 'nice'?" I asked.

"Well, that's one way to put it," said Donder. "She checks and rechecks her own checks! Then she eventually turns the list over to Santa, who rechecks *her* checks. It's a lot of responsibility for one Reindeer."

I shuddered. That's one job I was glad not to have!

"Anyway," continued Donder, "Santa has come to trust her judgment over the last 1,100 years."

"Could I go and see the operation now?" I asked excitedly.

"All right, let's go take a look!" Donder agreed.

We went outside, and took a well-worn path that led to a large building trimmed in snowflake design and painted light blue. We heard melodies floating out from inside. "It must be a happy place," I thought.

Donder opened the door and we stepped in. The place was alive with hustle and bustle. Elves carrying packages and mailsacks rushed by us, singing. A big circular desk sat in the center of the room—and Vixen sat behind it, wearing a green visor cap and with a pencil stuck behind her ear!

To one side of us were thousands of little mail cubby-holes covering a whole wall. There was a series of gliding ladders that rose from the floor to the ceiling. On each ladder were perched twenty or so elves, sorting mail and singing.

It seemed to be both a careful and a cheerful operation. I watched Vixen as she carefully read and checked several letters. When she was sure which slot one belonged in, she would deftly throw it across the room, where it would land neatly in her chosen target.

I was amazed! Letters were flying everywhere across the room. Vixen's circular desk also held a number of computer terminals. Every now and then, she would turn to one and use the keyboard with her front hooves. I could hear her say, "Southern Hemisphere, 86 degrees, Southeastern Seaboard, due south, north by northwest, longitude 27 degrees north..." I was fascinated by her total and complete control over the North Pole mailroom.

Some more elves came through the side doors loaded down with mailbags filled with yet more letters. Vixen waved them to the far side of the room where they dumped out the sacks' contents.

The letters were fed down a conveyor belt that ran the entire length of the building. Elves were packed in front of the belt, and they would grab letters off of it, glance at them, and throw them across the room into a kind of mail chute. These letters went straight to Vixen, who scooped them up and examined each one.

Suddenly the singing began to grow stronger, and soon the elves were tapping their feet to the music. Vixen looked up as she sorted mail, and also began to dance to the music. It was fantastic to watch her as she would dance and throw, never missing her target!

How she could keep up with all of this was beyond me!

"Can I talk to her while she's doing that?" I asked.

"Go ahead and talk, Lad," encouraged Vixen. "I'm used to doing several things at once."

"Vixen," I asked, "how in the world can you keep

up with all of this mail and know exactly which slot each and every letter belongs in?"

Vixen grinned and explained, "It's a matter of concentration, Lad." She sat down again in her chair and started rolling around as she worked, still tossing letters. She gave some orders to several elves next to the sliding ladders. "Don't you just love the atmosphere in here?" she asked.

Donder shouted over the singing, "*Can you come over to Grandfather Blitzen's house tonight around 6:00?*"

"Sure," she yelled. "Be through here around 4:30. See you then."

As we left Donder said, "Now you know why I don't want anything to do with the mailroom! But Vixen loves it. She says it relaxes her—and she feels needed. It's a most important operation.

More elves trooped by us, carrying still more stacks of mail. On the wall across from the mail-slots was a large list, simply labeled "NAUGHTY" and "NICE."

I noticed that there weren't any names yet on the "Naughty" list, and I pointed this out to Donder.

"Well, for one thing, many of the letters are thank-yous this time of year. And, as I told you, she won't put many names on the naughty list anyway. If she does, she always goes over them with Santa first."

Donder nudged me and I looked up. I gasped! Suddenly the whole room looked like a snowstorm was raging inside! There were literally thousands of letters flying through the air. It was just Santa's Christmas mailroom in full operation.

Donder showed me one more detail, as he poked me to get my attention and pointed to the ceiling. High above us, elves were swinging from ropes that had been tied around their middles. Across the room they'd swing to grab a handful of mail, then swing back and put the letters in their rightful slots. Other elves standing on the floor handed them the bundles of letters—and the process went on and on. No one was standing still for a minute!

Glancing at Vixen before we left, I saw her standing on top of her desk throwing mail with her front hooves.

Elves kept dumping sacks of mail on her desk, and emptying the bags of letters in front of her. She would kneel quickly, grab a handful, and continue the furious sorting!

Donder said as he opened the door, "She's on a roll now. The elves love her. She's the best there's ever been at sorting world mail and keeping up with everything and everyone. No one else would want to run the mailroom, but she keeps it in good order, year after year!"

"How long does this go on?" I asked, still amazed.

"Just about year 'round. It'll slow down for a week or two at a time, and then pick up again. Vixen wouldn't miss it for the world. She loves her work!"

Finally we reached Donder's home. As we went inside, he said he would make us some sandwiches. I went to my desk and started sorting out all the notes I had taken for the day. I didn't want to forget anything I had seen—how could I *ever* forget such sights and sounds, anyway!

15

The Christmas Jobs of Dasher and Comet

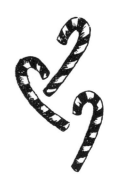

Donder called me from the kitchen to inform me that lunch was ready. I sat down at the table for a healthful meal.

"After we eat," he suggested, "we can rest for an hour or so and then talk some more about the interviews you have yet to schedule. Or we can go down to the fabric department and see what Comet and Dasher are doing."

I was too excited about my assignment to do much resting. "Let's go watch Comet and Dasher," I chose. "What was it exactly that Santa wanted them to do?"

"They're in charge of the production of all stuffed animals—deciding what color eyes, tails, fur—everything that makes up a complete toy."

"Sounds like fun. Let's go!" I responded.

We walked down the snowy path that I was becoming pretty familiar with by now. We turned right at Santa's castle, and Donder pointed out the large building with multicolored stained glass windows where Dasher and Comet worked. It was painted frosty, light gray, with big, blue icicles hanging all along the outside eves. On the outside walls were painted colorful depictions of teddy bears, lions, tigers, puppies, cats, and other animals. I could hear music coming from the inside of this building, too, as we neared the big double doors and entered.

"Are there many elves working here?" I asked. Suddenly, before he could answer, I saw what looked like elves' feet scurrying past us—I couldn't see anything but their feet since their bodies were hidden by the biggest panda bears I had ever seen! They were taking the bears into a little side room.

"Final processing," said Donder, as we walked across the floor, where we saw Dasher sitting on a high-backed stool almost in the center of the big room. An endless procession of elves was walking by in front of him, each carrying a stuffed animal toy. The elves would pause for just an instant, and Dasher would tell each what the animal needed for completion.

"Long, fuzzy tail, short ears, color—brown..." I saw Dasher grimace slightly as the next elf stepped up in front of him. "Oh, don't hold him like that! All the stuffing will rush to his head. That's right, color—bright red."

Dasher would stop every so often and bend down to touch a stuffed toy gently. "He has to get the feel of them," explained Donder.

Suddenly Dasher turned and saw us. "BREAAK!" he announced to his fellow-workers.

As the elves scurried to the hot chocolate and cookie table, Dasher walked with us there too. "Well, what do you think of the stuffed animal toy department, Lad?"

I grinned. "I think it's neat. How many animals do you see in a day's time?"

Dasher thought for a moment and then said,

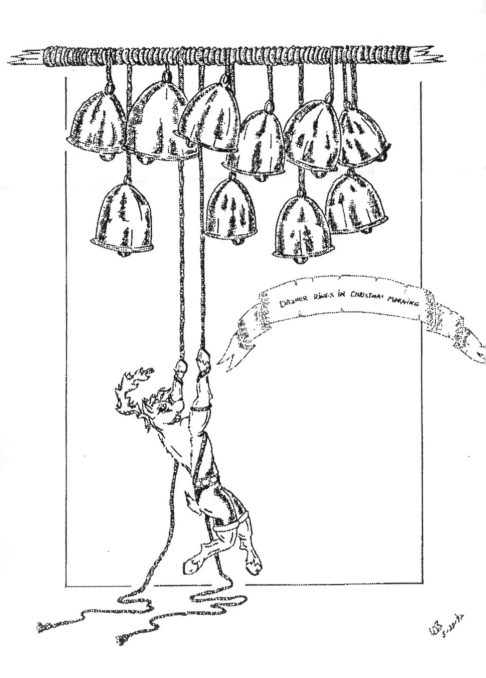

"From six to seven thousand. And they all have to be just right. Can't have any mixups, or you might invent a new animal!"

There were stuffed animals everywhere. Sitting against walls, on shelves and tables, piled on top of each other. Rabbits in one corner, elephants in another. And teddy bears of all shapes and colors and sizes—all cute and lovable as the next.

He explained how each stuffed animal toy had to have his or her own personality. Some of the toys were much bigger than the elves that carried them. Giant teddy bears walked by, followed by cute little raccoons and rabbits, chipmunks, squirrels, birds, and more teddy bears! I was starting to get dizzy as the colors blurred past me. The music swelled, and I could have sworn that the animals themselves were alive and dancing to the rhythm.

Donder reached down and snatched up a big teddy bear, elf and all. He started dancing across the floor. The elf's feet were simply hanging beneath the teddy bear in the air, as his arms clenched tightly around the bear's middle. As Donder swung them around, I could see the elf was laughing with merriment. Finally he put down both elf and bear. "Comet's just in the other part of the building," he told us. "Let's go see him. You'll really get a kick out of what Comet does."

We walked across the big room and were about to go through a set of double swinging doors when Dasher screamed to us, "See you tonight at 6:00 at Blitzen's house!"

We waved back our agreement and went on to see Comet.

"Dasher really likes his job," said Donder. "He has

The Christmas Jobs of Dasher and Comet   153

always said that every animal and teddy bear has to be perfect, because you can't fool a child."

I was just going to ask if we could come back tomorrow, when we ran smack into the back of Santa Claus. Or rather, I did. I was almost on the floor, when two strong arms caught me and set me back upright again. It was Grandfather Blitzen.

"Well, Lad, what do you think of our North Pole operation so far?" asked Santa.

"It's fantastic! Everything is so organized, and everyone is so happy," I said excitedly.

"Aye," said Blitzen. "Suit the Reindeer or the elf to his work, and you have a happy company."

Santa took me by the arm and led me through the middle of this enormous room. I could see Comet in the center. He appeared to be moving smoothly through the crowd of elves. He waved, the elves parted, and Comet came gliding up to us. He was on roller skates!

"Comet, how are the orders coming?" Santa asked. "Have we caught up with that backlog yet?"

"Yes. In fact, we're 'way ahead of schedule. I was just about to call for a break."

Santa nodded his approval.

"Want to see what we do in here, Lad?" asked Comet.

"Sure do," I said.

Blitzen asked Donder, "Are we still on for tonight? No changes?"

"No changes. Everyone will be there at 6:00."

Blitzen nodded and turned back to Santa. Comet led me to a row of metal lockers and opened one. Inside were several pairs of skates, their wheels sparkling in the light.

"What size do you wear, Lad?" Comet asked.

"What, me?" I stammered.

I hadn't skated in years. But I heard myself replying "Size 10½, please."

Donder was already lacing up his own skates. I sat down beside him on a candy cane bench and took off my elf shoes. "Look, it's gonna be easier than you think," he assured me. "These are special twinkle skates."

Now I was really worried! What if my skates had a mind of their own? Donder stood up and was quickly wheeled away through the crowd. Then he whished back to stop neatly on a dime next to Comet and me.

Warily and shakily, I stood up and started my way slowly across the floor, my arms out at my sides for balance. I noticed some elves around me snickering.

Comet advised, "Let your arms down, Lad. Just relax. You won't fall. The twinkle skates won't let you."

I was skeptical. But all at once I felt both feet take off with a jerk, and I was sailing across the floor, headed right for the refreshment table where Santa and Blitzen stood. Any elves in my path quickly scattered.

I was sure I was going to ram right into Santa and Blitzen. I covered my face with my hands and started screaming, "LOOK OUT!"

Looking through my fingers, I saw the table just ahead. That was it, I thought. No more North Pole, no more Santa Claus and the Reindeer, no more elves! I was going to run smack into the Main Man up here and ruin everything!

Suddenly, something grabbed my arm and I was spun into a 180-degree turn, away from Santa and Blitzen. We zoomed across the floor toward a huge pile of teddy bears, all with outstretched arms. Comet turned me loose and I disappeared into the soft, plush toy pile. Some elves rushed to me and dug me out, but I refused to stand up. I didn't want the skates to take off—with me in them—again!

"Hey, that was great!" teased Comet. "Where did you learn to skate like that?"

Donder came to a stop beside Comet, grinning.

"That's right, guys, laugh it up! I almost creamed Santa straight-on and you two think it's a joke! Help me get these things off."

"Naw, just keep them on. It's all in knowing how they work. Don't try to control the skates themselves; they have stardust bearings in them. Just think where you want to go, and the twinkle skates will get you there."

"Right. Do they understand the word 'Stop'?" I asked skeptically.

"Sure," said Donder. "Just think 'Stop' and they will."

So I got up again and tried. The skates really did respond to my thoughts, so that I could control where I was going. I was even able to evade a collision with the living tidal wave of elves rushing back to their stations after the break was over.

So Comet led me, on my skates, over to a much larger room. The work in here went much faster. I noticed a conveyor belt that ran the entire length of the room, then around the corners, and back down the other side of the room. Elves were busy stitching and sewing the right color eyes onto each stuffed animal. Then the finished toy was carefully placed in its own Christmas box by some thirty elves standing at the end of the conveyor belt. The pace of their work was mind-boggling.

Comet suggested, "Here, Lad, you try it. Just lean in between the elves, glance at the stuffed animal, and then tell the elf what color the eyes should be. I'll follow you in case you need help."

So I tried. I leaned down to my first stuffed animal and saw that it was a giraffe, lightly cream-colored with brown spots. I told the elf, "Light brown eyes," and moved to the next elf. As I flew down the line, the elves would reach into a bigger box to their left and snatch out the glass eyes I described. This was fun! I was just starting my eighth round, when I noticed that Comet wasn't following me anymore.

I kept on, doing pretty well on my own. When Santa entered the room he remarked, "Very good, Lad, for a first-timer!" I beamed.

"It was fun," I admitted as we prepared to leave. "I'd love to do this every day."

"I wonder how you'd feel doing it every day for 1,700 years, Lad?" Donder asked, smiling at me.

Then he told me, "Now it's vitamin time. Every day Cupid makes the rounds of all the elves and Reindeer and pops a multivitamin into their mouths. It's her own concoction. She even coats them with honey to make them slide right down!"

As we went to put away the twinkle skates, Comet rolled by and Donder reminded him again about the 6:00 meeting at Grandfather Blitzen's.

We left the building then, stepping back into the cold air, and heading up the hill.

"Donder," I asked, "do you ever get tired of doing the same thing day after day? Year after year?"

"Never. We wouldn't be happy doing anything else. It's not so much that we do the same thing year after year—it's the thought of those we're doing it *for*.

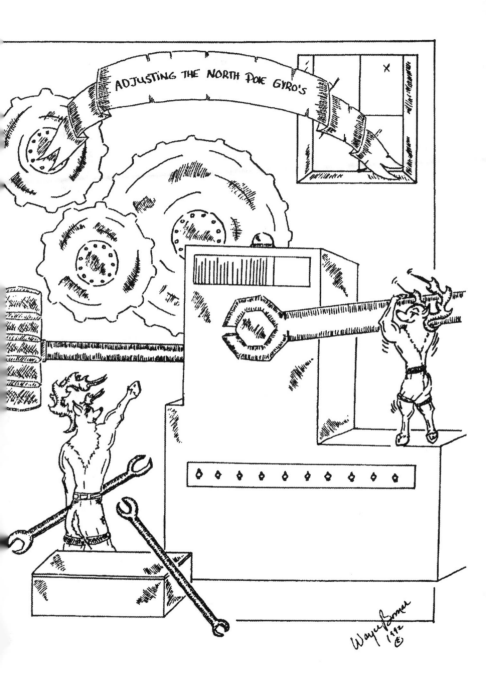

The children. That will never change. Did you see anyone in any department with a frown or a scowl?"

I had to admit I hadn't. It had been a blissfully fulfilling (if somewhat hectic) day.

We returned to Donder's house. Once inside, we flopped down on chairs in front of his fireplace. "Donder," I asked, "why is it that there's always a fire going in everyone's fireplace? Who tends them, anyway?"

"There's a special team of elves who see to it that each fireplace is kept going. They make the rounds of each home, stoke the fires, and leave enough wood outside on the porch to do the night. Since there's no dishonesty here, we all leave our doors open to them. They will also clean the hearths and sweep the chimneys if they need it. We leave special presents for the wood elves every Christmas Eve."

I thought awhile about labor, North Pole style. Here everyone had a job to do, and no one ever seemed to complain about doing too much. What a neat place! How I wished the rest of the world could be like that.

Donder sensed my thoughts and answered my unspoken words: "Me too, Lad... me too."

We sat and watched the fire a bit longer. I was really looking forward to our visit tonight with Grandfather Blitzen. Just the thought of the majestic, old Christmas Reindeer gave me a great feeling of security. I wondered how many times he had watched me as I slept, or as I waited for them all to arrive on Christmas Eve.

I couldn't wait to learn more answers to add to my book. I would write down the Reindeer's stories for the world to know.

We got ready for the evening quickly, and then left to walk to Blitzen's house. After we knocked at his front door, Comet answered and waved us in. I shivered with excitement as I thought of what was ahead.

16

An Evening at Grandfather Blitzen's

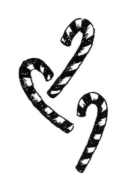

As we entered Grandfather Blitzen's house, I thought what a privilege it was to be invited to the home of the first-chosen Reindeer. He saw us in immediately, and invited us to sit around his enormous fireplace. Then he went into the kitchen, calling for Donder and Cupid to help him serve hot punch and his special chip wafers (considered a real treat among the Reindeer). They consist of flecks of chocolate, pecans and peanut butter, all fried up golden brown like little patties.

Donder and Cupid came back into the living room holding huge, flat trays of hot chip wafers. Sounds of *Hmmmm* filled the room. They set them down on a rather unusual-looking table, just in front of the hearth. Instead of having legs, it was supported by wood runners, varnished and waxed to match the top. I gently ran my hands over the finish, admiring the quality of workmanship, and helping myself to a chip wafer at the same time.

Grandfather Blitzen came back into the room then, holding a tray loaded with mugs of steaming punch. He sat down heavily on his easy chair. Turning to me, he said, "I noticed that ye were admiring the center table."

"It's beautiful," I said appreciatively, running my hand down its smooth top. "I have never seen anything like it."

"Aye, 'tis unique, Lad," he said. "The only one like it in all the world. 'Tis the very first Christmas sled that the good Santa Claus and I used. I had it finished just so when we retired it and started using the great sleigh. Did the varnish work myself. 'Tis a grand old table, and each crack and dent holds many memories for this old Reindeer! Aye!"

I was in awe. Grandfather Blitzen's home was most impressive. His Christmas tree especially was a thing of beauty. It must have been ten feet tall, and the star atop it was glowing gold and throwing out radiant beams.

Grandfather Blitzen had lit his pipe now. Yet, sniffing at the air, I was surprised at the absence of any tobacco smell. Neither Santa nor Blitzen used tobacco in any form, I discovered. "'Tis a special Reindeer concoction, Lad," Blitzen explained, reading my thoughts. "Grows only in the high mountains of northern Canada, near a town called Inuvik."

As we sat around the fire, Blitzen began to tell us of days of old, long vanished, but still alive in the heart of each Christmas Reindeer. He reminisced about what a time he had had trying to teach a very young Comet how to run on the songs of the winds... how he had taught Donder to stand straight and tall in the harness instead of slumping.

Donder grinned wryly as that point came up.

After a time of further chatting together, we sat down to a lovely meal. Afterwards, we all carried our empty plates into the kitchen.

There I saw that Dancer had put on an apron and

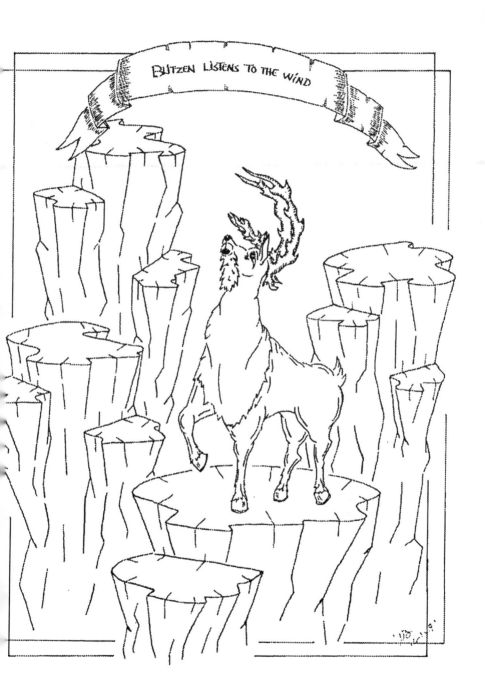

was washing the dirty dishes. I quickly grabbed another apron with a large Christmas tree on it and started drying.

"You don't have to do that, Lad," said Dancer, smiling, "you're our guest!"

"Guest or no guest, I'll do my share," I countered.

Just then Blitzen walked in. "Got you working, eh, Lad?"

"Oh, I don't mind, Grandfather," I said. "I enjoy everything I do here."

"Well, don't tarry too long," he warned. "I understand it's another story that ye'll be wanting to hear, Lad." And Blitzen winked at me.

When we were through with chores and once again settled by the fire, Dancer, leaning forward, said, "Won't you tell us the story of the misplaced Christmas Eve again?"

"Please tell it, Grandfather," agreed Cupid.

Blitzen, having gotten his ancient pipe going again, suddenly threw back his massive antlers and gave a hearty laugh.

"Aye, 'twas a Christmas Eve, that was!"

Blitzen pointed to a picture at one side of the mantelpiece. "Look close, Lad, and see if that reminds you of someone."

I recognized Grandfather Blitzen, but for the life of me I couldn't tell who it was he was holding in his arms. Could it be... *Cupid?*

She looked so small in his arms, and had such an impish grin on her face.

"Aye, Lad," he said, realizing I had guessed, "'tis little Elsker, no more than a year old. I had just caught her in the sweet cider in my storage shed."

Cupid blushed and lowered her head. "Grandfather!"

"I just knew he was going to spank me," she explained, "so I ran."

Blitzen chuckled. "Aye, Elsker ran like the wind. Took me nearly three miles to catch her!"

Blitzen then became thoughtful. "'Twas not a spanking that you needed, Little One. 'Twas the run! I didn't mind the small amount of cider you took. 'Twas your spirit that gladdened me. Deep within, I knew ye knew right from wrong—so I didn't have the heart to scold ye."

Then, at once, with a sweep of his arm, Blitzen began the real story.

"'Twas a cold night *that* Christmas Eve! And a very busy night. The year had been more hectic than any I remember. Elves were everywhere, scurrying and scampering. The load of toys on the great sleigh was massive. Never had I, in my long life, seen such a load!

"The sleigh fairly swayed with the enormous weight. Everyone was singing carols, and it made my old heart glad to be a part of it all. Such was the Christmas spirit that year.

"I had already made the decision that topcoats would be worn under the harness that year, it was so very cold! Santa was busy checking this and that. Mrs. Claus was all abustle, loading snacks for us all into the great sleigh. The stars were twinkling brightly, and the sky was a cold, clear mirror.

"The line from the Great Hall of Elves was something to see—elves lined up in two rows passing gifts and toys to each other up the rows—all to be put into the sleigh.

"It seemed we were running slightly behind schedule, and everyone was working extra hard to get us off. At last, every toy was loaded, and Cupid, having hitched us in securely, made ready herself.

"The door to Santa's house opened, and out came the good Santa Claus, looking grand in his traditional red. He was slapping his white-mittened hands together to keep them warm, and he breathed out great clouds of white frost.

"If I remember correctly, that was also the night that a very young Dancer had rolled one of the elves into a big snowball. But that was nothing compared to the time Dancer had some of the elves believing they could fly like us! They were jumping out of the loft window, arms outstretched and flapping wildly—landing, fortunately, in a big snowdrift... Aye! But that's another story..."

Blitzen almost got sidetracked. He thought for a moment and then continued: "Santa had climbed aboard the great sleigh. And just as he picked up the reins and started to yell, 'Away, Blitzen, away!' he was stopped by his chief elf, Newton—who came running up, all out of breath, yelling 'STOP!'

"Santa put down the reins and looked in Newton's direction, holding onto the side of the sleigh as though to hold it fast to the ground. 'Santa!' the elf called hoarsely. 'There's been a terrible mistake."

"'What do you mean, Newton? Everything's in order. The toys are loaded, my Reindeer are hitched in and ready to go. What could be wrong?'

"Newton looked terribly uncomfortable. He leaned up to Santa and whispered something in his ear. Santa looked stunned, as though in a trance. He got up quickly from the sleigh and walked toward his house.

"Summoning Newton to the front of the team, I asked him what could possibly have happened. He told me shakily that we had used the wrong calendar! 'Tonight is actually the 23rd of December,' he announced sadly.

We were ahead of ourselves by one calendar day. *The next day* was actually Christmas Eve!"

I was so engrossed in Grandfather Blitzen's tale that I jumped up, screaming, *"What on earth did you do?"*

Blitzen chuckled and said, "Well, needless to say, Lad, everyone became totally deflated at hearing about the mixup. We figured the only thing we could do was go home and wait until tomorrow. Cupid began to unhitch everyone. But then we all heard a curious sort of humming coming from Dancer. We all knew that sound. He was computing mathematical equations in his mind at a terrific rate. Suddenly he stopped humming and yelled, *'Wait, everyone!* Get Santa back here. Quickly!!!'

"Then Dancer went back to humming again. Thinking that it might be another one of his jokes, I almost told him to stop. But Vixen grabbed my arm and whispered urgently, 'Wait! Wait, Grandfather Blitzen. Dancer's serious.'

"By now he had closed his eyes tightly and looked like he was far away. Santa came up and stood beside us then. He had already changed into more casual clothes. He looked pretty annoyed as he asked, 'Well, what is it?'

"Dancer suddenly spoke from out of his 'trance.' *'South, due south—0 degrees longitude—a complete circle. Fifteen minutes, earth time, traveling in the upper atmosphere at a height of 3.6 miles...'"*

"Santa rubbed his hands through his hair, and, staring at me, said, 'What's he talking about?'"

At this point, Blitzen chuckled and puffed on his pipe. Looking at Dancer and smiling, he said, "I hadn't the faintest idea what he meant, and was about to say so—when Donder figured out what Dancer had been doing. He tried to explain to Santa:

"'Santa, Dancer says that if we fly due south on a 0 degree heading 3.6 miles high in the upper stratosphere, that in 15 minutes, when we land back here, it will be December 24th, CHRISTMAS EVE!'

"'How is that possible?' asked Santa, scratching his head.

"Dancer then started explaining to us a series of complicated mathematical equations concerning space-time continuum displacement. It was really getting deep, when Newton, who had been figuring right along with Dancer, became animated and started to jump around shouting, 'He's right! By the Great Star, Dancer's right!'

"Cupid was already starting to hook up the traces again as we all took our places. Santa paused for a long moment, covering his eyes and drawing what looked like figures in the air in front of him. For several minutes he did that, 'erasing' them, and then 'drawing' them again. Then he lit up like a lightbulb and announced: 'Hook up the Reindeer. Load up the sleigh... we're losing time. We must away!!!'

"Everything was as it had been before we realized our mistake. The spirit, the singing, the laughter. Santa ran back to his house to change. Then, jumping into the sleigh, he grabbed the reins and shouted for the takeoff. Newton crouched outside the sleigh beside Santa with a stopwatch in his hand, as we all grabbed the wind turbulence at the end of the icy runway and lifted off.

"And it was just as Dancer had figured. Along the stratosphere we flew with the speed of a red-hot bullet. Dancer held us all to a true course of 0 degrees. Inside of 15 minutes, we again touched down at the North Pole, having circled the earth. *The time was December 24th!* Christmas Eve! I do believe Dancer's head became almost too tight for his muzzle straps that night, he swelled so with pride. But we had to admit, if it hadn't been for him, we would have had to wait an extra day!"

Blitzen began to tamp his pipe. Everyone was laughing, and Comet and Dasher were pounding Dancer on the back. I thought it was a grand tale. And, better yet, it was *true!*

After we had all laughed and hugged each other following this exciting recollection—we quieted down once again. We knew that, next, Grandfather Blitzen was going to tell the story of how Vixen had become a Christmas Reindeer. I turned to a clean page of my notepad, switched on my tape recorder, and awaited another magical tale.

17

A Christmas Reindeer Named Vixen

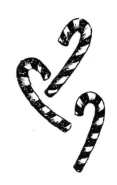

Grandfather Blitzen looked around the room at his beloved fellow Christmas Reindeer. "The best place to start is at the beginning," he said. "Her true name is... Anna."

I heard Vixen give a start, and I saw that she had placed her hooves above her mouth and was staring at Grandfather Blitzen. She looked surprised. I realized then that she had had no idea that tonight was planned as the time for Blitzen to recount her story.

Vixen stuttered, "Grandfather, must you? I'll be so embarrassed." She hid her face again with her hooves.

Blitzen smiled, and reaching over, gently touched Vixen on her cheek and whispered, "Nonsense, Anna. Your chronicle is filled with great love. Lad must know how each of us came to be Christmas Reindeer."

Vixen looked up and nodded, "Very well, Grandfather. I'll just go and get everyone some more hot punch." And she quickly got up and went into the kitchen.

Dasher quietly chuckled. "Isn't that just like Vixen? She's the first to scold us when we act up, but also the first to put her own story off as nothing."

I turned back to Grandfather Blitzen, who was

puffing on his pipe, collecting his thoughts. Finally he began to tell this wonderful story of love.

"Unlike some of you, Anna had to fend for herself when she was very young. Her homeland was torn apart by war. Anna lived from day to day, never knowing if it would be her last. She was strong... she had to be. But she was also kind and gentle, and filled with love.

"Anna wandered everywhere, but lived nowhere. Her birthplace was in the small town of Archangel, Russia, near the border of Finland. She really had no place to call home for many years. Everywhere she went, there was turmoil and confusion. She hid in the daylight and roamed at night. Anna always tried to help her people as best she could—tending to the sick, caring for the young and the elderly. It was during one Christmas Eve flight that we found her letter to us."

Blitzen smiled at Dasher. "Actually, it was Dasher who saw it and brought it to me. I read it, then brought it to the attention of the good Santa Claus. Anna had left us a letter, written in desperation—not knowing if we would even come this way during our Christmas Eve flight.

"Fortunately, we did. Her letter was found outside one of the small houses, tacked to a tree. It asked simply that, if it were possible, would we help the cold and hungry children, since food was very scarce. She said that she had believed in the good Santa Claus and his magical Reindeer all of her life. *'Please, oh, please, leave food for the children!'*"

Blitzen wiped his eyes momentarily. Then, looking back up, he continued. "How could anyone's heart not be touched by such a letter?"

Just then, Vixen came back into the living room with a tray of hot drinks for everyone. As she served them, Grandfather Blitzen went on. "It was Dasher, Dancer, and Prancer who begged to leave the sleigh and go for food. We continued on our journey without them, agreeing to rendezvous with them near Paris, France, in a short time. Meeting them as we had planned, they told us of Anna—how she had been waiting for them, and how strong was her faith. Dasher described her as devoted, more than anything, to the children and their welfare.

"Yet she had looked haggard and weary, and her eyes betrayed the fear she lived with every day. Anna took the food and disappeared into the darkness, they said. But before she left them, she gave them a message for Santa.

"The letter said: 'To the good Santa Claus and his loyal Christmas Reindeer. It is with all my heart that I thank you for the gift of food for the children. The hard times in my country will pass, but forever across the magical skies of Christmas you shall all continue. I have seen you with my own eyes, and my work will be easier from this day on. I shall live for the children of all countries, for this you have taught me through the generosity of giving.'"

Blitzen gently patted Vixen's knee as she sat beside him, her head bowed, her eyes moist with remembrance. Cupid put her arm around Vixen's shoulder and held her tightly, and Donder got up to stand behind her, gently putting his front hooves on her shoulders also.

Blitzen relit his pipe and picked up the story of Anna. "We continued to receive Anna's letters each Christmas, asking for nothing for herself, but only for the children. The strife and turmoil finally ended in her land, but still she wrote to us. We found out from her that there were poor children who had no knowledge of Santa Claus! So each year we left for them what she asked for. We always left it in the same place, in a small abbey in the village of Archangel. She would gather the large bundles on her small back and then go and distribute the goods among the poor.

"Anna left gifts on doorsteps, anywhere she knew the children would find them. In a sense, she was helping us locate the children who had no way of letting us know what they wished for. Anna always made sure the gifts were signed: 'From Sinta Klauss and his Reindeer of love.'

"She brought so much joy and happiness to so many children, that it wasn't long before her legend—and her fame—began to grow. There were tales of a lone Reindeer trudging through deep snows with enormous bundles strapped to her frail back. Of course, no one ever saw this Reindeer bearing gifts for the children. But always, on Christmas morning, there would be presents on every doorstep, throughout the small villages. Why didn't we deliver gifts to these homes? you might ask. Well, this was Anna's calling.

"Thus she carried out her 'mission,' and she served in the best way she knew how: with love and devotion. She often worked long nights, and she never let anyone be forgotten.

"Oh, I kept watch over her throughout the years, and they were long years, for a mortal reindeer. Anna never missed a Christmas Eve.

"Then, on Christmas Eve in the Year of Our Lord 920, as we unloaded the great sleigh with the gifts she had asked for—she didn't come. We waited a long

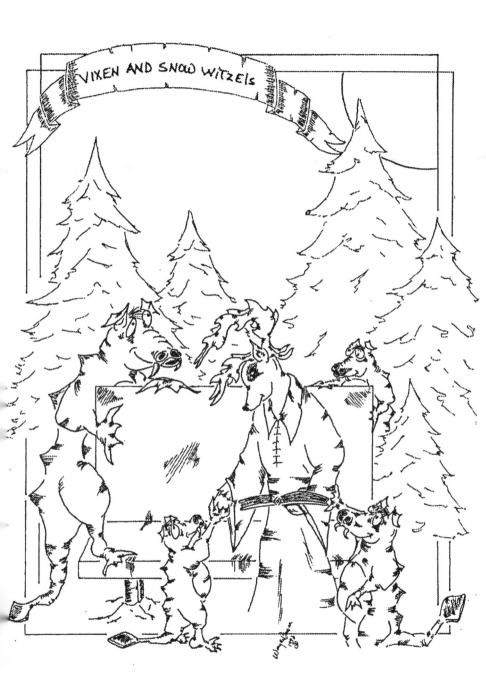

time, even searching the forest around the small abbey—but we couldn't find her."

I looked at Grandfather Blitzen and saw a single, silver tear trickle down his gray muzzle. "A terrible feeling of dread came over me, and so Dasher, Dancer, Prancer, Comet, and I took leave of the sleigh to go look for her. Donder used all his strength to finish the journey that Christmas Eve, pulling Santa and the sleigh by himself. He vowed that they would return when the other deliveries had been made—and they did. Then they began to help us go in search of Anna.

"We had all but given up hope of ever finding her, fearing the worst, when we heard Santa Claus calling to us from very far away to bring the great sleigh to him. So we pulled it, in search of his voice. A Christmas Reindeer can always hear the voice of Santa Claus calling to his 'children.'

"Up hills and down, Dancer followed Santa's voice. He finally led us to a very rugged part of the forest, where there stood a ramshackle lean-to, made from the branches of evergreen trees. Here we found Santa leaning over Anna, whispering softly in her ear. As we gathered around the lean-to, we saw that Anna was very, very sick.

"Her tracks in the deep snow told us that she had tried valiantly to reach the abbey, but so sick was she, that she simply could not make it. Anna had fallen many times in the cold, deep snow, but had managed to pull herself back to that squalid lean-to, where she had written what she had thought would be her last letter to us."

I found myself crying softly as the story continued. I saw Blitzen pull an old, yellowed letter from his vest pocket. Carefully unfolding it, he read it to us: "Good

Sinta Klauss, O wonderful and magical Reindeer of Christmas. I can go on no longer. Please deliver the gifts to my children..."

He looked at us, carefully put the letter away, took a deep breath, and said: "The letter was held by her front hoof, close to her heart. Santa Claus moved quickly, gathering her limp form up in his big arms. He quickly carried Anna to the great sleigh, lying her gently on the seat, and covered her with warm blankets. He used his red hat for her pillow. As we stood by, we saw that Anna's breath was very shallow. We all cried, not knowing what to do for her.

"Santa came to us, raised both hands to the heavens, and proclaimed urgently: 'She has given everything she had to give. We must act quickly before we lose her. The Beams of Immortality must shine on this precious creature of love if she is going to continue to live among us.' And then he implored the heavens, 'Be there one among ye Christmas Immortals who will stand for this creature of great self-sacrifice and devoted love?'

"Santa was reciting the Oath of Immortality that all of us had pledged when we became Christmas Reindeer. If one of the Christmas Immortals questions the oath, the ritual is in vain, and immortality beyond reach. Each one of us stood forth and quickly pledged ourselves for the life of Anna.

"Stepping up to the great sleigh, Santa turned to us and boomed, 'So be it! I, too, pledge myself for this courageous creature who has given everything she has to the children. She is to become one of us if we can but make it in time. The curtains of the Beams of Immortality have been opened but for a brief moment in time. Fly, my children, fly as you have never flown before! And pull with great love in your hearts, my immortal Christmas Reindeer—for the very life of Anna depends on it!'

"I knew then what Santa had done. If we could but make it through the curtains of the Beams of Immortality in time, Anna was to become a Christmas Reindeer. All of us quickly jumped into harness, and with a great heave, we leaped skyward, toward the far North.

"We all knew that a very short time remained for Anna. Santa laid her head in his lap and frantically urged us on. We strained with speed as we had never strained before. And we could feel Anna's life-force draining from her even as we progressed.

"We were all glowing with Christmas energy in our quest—like a shooting star in the dark night. Then, suddenly, far ahead of us, we could see the blanket beams that marked the boundary of Christmas immortality. That pushed us to even greater speeds. With a final effort, we entered the magical beams and were bathed in their warm, golden light. All of us felt the pure energy force enter Anna. For a while, we flew aimlessly in the beams of blessed purity. Anna, who had come so close to leaving us, raised her head ever so slightly.

"We all knew, then, that Anna had received a Christmas miracle. A startling transformation had taken place. Anna was no longer old. She was now a young, vibrant Christmas Reindeer. As suddenly as the beams had come, they vanished, and we were once again in the cold night sky.

"Slowly we turned toward the Great Star that beckoned us home. It was many days before Anna regained full consciousness, for the Beams of Immortality leave one stunned at first. When she did fully awake, we were there beside her.

"Anna opened her eyes slowly, and the first thing she said was, 'My children! Did you see how they smiled when they opened the gifts you brought?' Santa leaned close to her and whispered that she would never have to worry about her children again. She would be able to see to them personally every Christmas Eve.

"Anna's eyes opened wide at Santa's words, and, propping herself up, she looked at us with wonder and asked, 'Where am I?'"

Donder spoke now, as he held Vixen, who was still crying softly and swaying from side to side. "It was Grandfather Blitzen who knelt down and held her and said, 'You're one of us now, little Anna. Aye! You are a Christmas Reindeer, and you will journey with us throughout eternal Christmastime, now and forever.'

"It took her a while to fully realize the priceless gift she had been given. When she did understand, she wept with great joy. She marveled to again have a lithe, young body, full of energy. And, as you know, Lad, Anna has been with us since the year 921, and has continued to give of herself tirelessly. She has brought us great unity, and that oneness continues to grow among us. That is why she works in the mailroom—so that she can personally see to it that no child is ever passed over."

The room was silent for a few minutes. We all honored the life history—and the living legacy—of the Christmas Reindeer now known as Vixen.

18

A Trip to Iceland

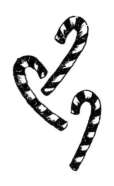

Donder and I turned in late that night. I sat up at my desk putting the finishing touches on the story of Vixen. Donder sat in front of the fire and dozed from time to time. It was well after 2:00 A.M. when I finally roused him and got him off to bed. Then I got into my own bed and was asleep at once.

During the night, I dreamed I was flying with the Christmas Reindeer as they made their trip around the world on Christmas Eve. The big bell atop the Great Hall of Toys woke me from a most pleasant scene. I roused myself reluctantly.

Donder stood at the door. He shook his big antlers and managed a morning grin, which was somewhat lopsided. "How about flapjacks?" he asked.

"Sounds great to me."

When we sat down in the kitchen for breakfast, I asked Donder: "What's on the schedule for today?"

Donder looked amused. He said, "Today, my young fellow, we are going to fly over to the island of Iceland."

My eyes widened. "Iceland? Why do we need to go to Iceland?"

Donder walked to the door and started putting on his antler coverings. I knew that meant one thing: high flying in cold altitudes.

"Donder," I begged, "please tell me *why* we need to go to Iceland."

"Because Grandfather Blitzen is sending us on a mission of greatest importance. We are going to get Dasher a birthday present."

"Birthday present?" I said. "When is Dasher's birthday?"

Donder stepped outside. I followed, grabbing my topcoat, buttoning it, and wrapping a scarf around my neck.

"Tomorrow is Dasher's birthday. We always throw a big party for anyone's birthday, and Dasher is no exception. Grandfather Blitzen wants the present this year to be very special.

"Iceland is Dasher's homeland. We will go to Husavik, his hometown, and shop around for something suitable."

I hurried behind Donder. He was headed for the great sleigh's storage shed, I presumed to get a saddle for me, as Comet had done when I rode with him to get the blue ice.

I assumed wrong. Donder, with my help, pulled an ancient-looking sled down from its rack on the wall. He began hitching a single harness rig to it.

"Why don't we just fly, Donder?" I asked.

Donder grinned and said, "It would look kinda funny, don't you think, if I just came flying into town with you riding on my back?"

I guess he was right—but I was wary of that sled. I had never ridden on one of these small ones before.

Donder finished hooking his harness onto the sled. Then he turned to me and said, "Not to worry, Lad. All you have to do is sit here. I'll do the rest."

The sled really didn't look very stable, as I climbed

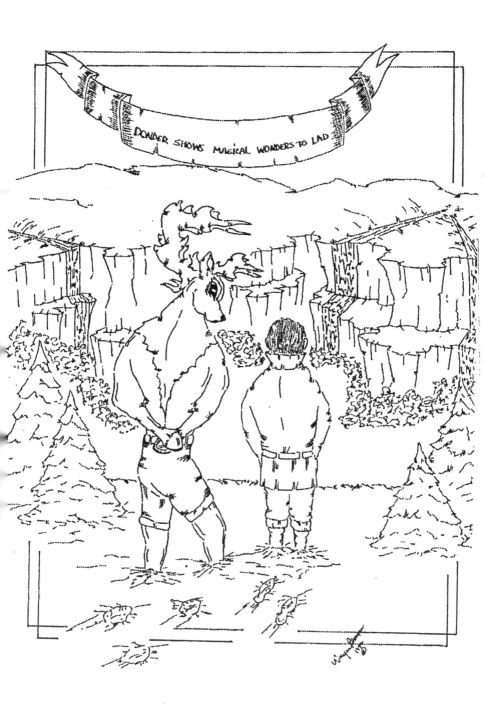

aboard and gripped the sides. Donder slipped the harness over his big shoulders and asked, "Ready?" I nodded my head. I guess I was ready for just about anything.

Donder turned toward the open door of the shed and, digging in with his powerful back legs, took off running. The sled was jerking around terribly. I was holding onto the sides fervently!

He made a 90-degree turn in front of the Great Hall of Toys, just as Dasher, Comet, and Prancer stepped out of the big double doors. They all waved as we went *whooshing* by. I tried to wave back, but my teeth were rattling so hard, I couldn't manage much of a wave! I did see that they were all laughing.

I must have looked like a rubber ball, the way I was bouncing around on the sled as he pulled it on ground. Donder was headed for a very steep hill. VERY steep! It wasn't the steepness that bothered me so much—it was the fact that the hill seemed to have no bottom, but instead led down to a yawning abyss! Donder picked up speed as he fairly rocketed down the hill—or cliff! I was scared speechless as the edge of the abyss rushed toward us. Donder was showing no signs of taking to the air.

I opened my mouth to scream, when I suddenly felt the sled give a jerk, and Donder really dug in with his back feet. We were airborne! We had just cleared the top of the cliff! I was looking over the edge of the sled straight down perhaps a mile. The sled was pretty stable now, so I tried to calm down and enjoy the ride.

Donder began to climb. He was indeed a magnificent sight as he ran the wind-currents. He held his head high, tasting the freshness of the air, and sniffing the wind as it rushed by us. I could tell that Donder really enjoyed flying. He, like Comet, would stretch his front legs 'way out in front of him, with his back legs tucked beneath him. Then he would push off with his front legs, and tuck *them* beneath him.

We circled the compound below us, and I could still see Dasher, Comet, and Prancer standing there where I had last seen them. They were waving at us. Feeling better than the last time we had passed them, I waved wildly back at them. Vixen and Cupid had also joined them now. "See you all later," I shouted.

Donder, with a great heave of his back legs, banked sharply to the right and headed toward open country, still climbing. I sat on my little perch of a sled and watched this Christmas Reindeer thoroughly enjoying himself.

Apparently, we were in no hurry. Just under the small seat of the sled was a picnic basket that Grandfather Blitzen had packed our lunch in. I was glad I had worn my heavy topcoat, as the blue sky was starting to fade to darkness. I dared to look down—something I had told myself I wouldn't do.

Just then Donder yelled back to me, *"Greenland!"* I saw the beautiful coast of that land once again and wondered if we were anywhere near where Comet and I had been so recently. We flew along the coast of the Greenland Sea. If I remembered my geography correctly, Iceland would be the next large land-mass we would see. For about an hour we flew lazily along, just enjoying the view.

Then Donder began to descend. Looking ahead, I could just make out several hot water geysers ahead of us. They spewed scalding water hundreds of feet in the air. Donder landed the sled—and me—just to the side of one of these spectacular wonders of nature.

He grabbed the picnic basket from under the seat, having quickly slipped his traces. "Let's eat, I'm starving," he said, leading me to a small, grassy knoll that overlooked the geysers.

We had an excellent lunch of Blitzen's famous chip wafers and fried moss sandwiches—a Reindeer specialty. Some fruit and then fig newtons—my favorite—topped off the meal. The Reindeer really did know all about me!

Donder also found a note from Blitzen, under the napkins. It read: "Now, boys, don't tarry too long in the land of midnight sun. After you've eaten, go straight to Husavik and pick up Dasher's present. And Donder—*no talking* while you're there. I don't want to have to go and get you out of some zoo!" We had a good laugh over that advice.

We got up to resume our journey. "Well, let's get a move on," Donder said. "Even though I CAN maintain an air speed of Mach 7. We're burning daylight, as John Wayne used to say!"

I had no more than sat down in the sled, when Donder was off with a jerk that sent us both hurtling straight up. I had just tucked the picnic basket under the seat when Donder yelled, "Iceland! Straight ahead!"

Donder swerved to the left and followed the coastline of Iceland. Across the Denmark Strait we flew, while Donder closely scanned the coastline. Suddenly, with a sharp bank to the right, we dove straight down. Donder leveled out, and just ahead I could see a small village.

We landed on the outskirts. I quickly got out of the sled and we prepared to go into town. He slipped his head through a loop in the rope I held. It seemed so strange leading him as he pulled the sled— realizing he was one of Santa's magical Christmas Reindeer!

We went from shop to shop. I couldn't understand a word of what people were saying, since it was all in Icelandic.

Donder would whisper a translation to me from time to time. We finally chose a gift for Dasher: a beautiful handcarved woodcutting that portrayed the people of Husavik working on their fishing boats.

As the shopkeeper carefully wrapped the carving for me, I suddenly remembered that I didn't have any money! When the man held his hand out for the payment, I stood there frozen, not knowing what to do.

Donder nudged me. I looked at him, and he swung his head toward the sled. I didn't know what he meant. Finally, he hissed, "The basket, Lad, look in the basket!" The man behind the counter leaned over and looked at us both, quite puzzled.

"He's got the sniffles," I explained. He had no idea what I had said, anyway.

I went out to the sled and pulled out the picnic basket. There in the bottom was a wooden box which held several coins. I gave them to the man and received the wood carving.

We had done it—we'd gotten just the right gift for Dasher!

Donder once again slipped into the harness of the sled. Just as we were about to take off, I heard shouts behind us. Donder and I turned to see five or six men running toward us, followed by twenty or thirty children. They were all shouting excitedly, "Sinta Klauss …Sinta Klauss!"

Donder said, "Oh, oh!" and took off with a powerful push. We flew directly over the heads of the men and children, as the children squealed and danced with delight.

I felt pretty good, having been mistaken for Santa Claus!

"They'll talk about this for years to come," said Donder. "How one day Santa and one of his Reindeer came to their village and bought a wood carving."

We both laughed happily, and Donder turned toward home.

Donder made good time, and within a few hours we were again at the North Pole. We landed in front of the storage shed. After pushing the sled back onto its rack, we walked back outside and up the hill toward the Reindeer compound.

"Man, what a day! I'm famished," said Donder.

I held the wrapped woodcutting under my arm. As we started across the big circle compound with the big Christmas tree in the center, we ran into Grandfather Blitzen. "Did ye get a nice gift for Dasher?" he asked.

Donder nodded his head and smiled. "The best yet, Grandfather. I think he'll really enjoy it, don't you, Lad?"

"Oh, yes," I agreed. "Dasher will absolutely love it."

Blitzen nodded his head and walked away. We heard him say under his breath: "And some children got the thrill of thinking they saw Santa up close!"

"How'd he know?" I asked Donder as we watched the old Reindeer walk off down the hill.

Donder just shrugged his shoulders. "How does Grandfather Blitzen know everything that goes on around here and... the world?"

We turned toward Donder's house. Once inside, we hit the easy chairs for some hard-earned moments of dozing!

19

Dasher's Birthday and His Great Speed

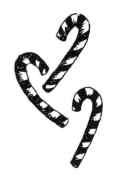

We didn't know it at the time, but those "moments" of dozing were to last the whole night. Early the next morning, Donder nudged me. When I opened my eyes, he said, "Man, that sure was an exhausting trip yesterday! We both overslept."

Hurriedly we ate the breakfast he had prepared: french toast with Vermont maple syrup. Today, I just remembered, was Dasher's birthday!

It was going to be a great day!

We wrapped the wood carving carefully, and got ready to set out. Donder explained that all birthday parties were held in the Great Hall of Toys.

When we got there, Vixen met us at the door and said, "Dancer has taken Dasher on a phony medical run. They should be gone about three hours."

"Where did you tell Dasher he was going this time?" asked Donder, chuckling.

Vixen looked at me and explained. "Every year on Dasher's birthday, one of us will tell him he is needed for a fast medical run. After about 300 years of doing this to him, always on his birthday, Dasher is wise to it, of course. He knows it's just an excuse to get him away from the North Pole while we decorate the Hall for his party. But he cooperates anyway."

Vixen giggled. "This time, Dancer and Dasher are headed for Peru. Even though Dancer is quite convincing (as you know!)—Dasher wasn't buying it for a minute. But he went along with it to be a good sport."

"It's been worse in other years. Dasher got really tired of flying around in circles about 40 years ago on his birthday. Dancer had told him he forgot where they were going, and kept him circling until he could recover his 'memory'! It took Dasher about 30 minutes to leave that nonsense and return to the Pole—and Dancer two hours!"

Donder continued, chuckling, "Dasher was really moving on when he hit the lower atmosphere over the Pole. We all heard the sonic boom when he broke the sound barrier. Dasher's speed was officially recorded that day as just over Mach 8. Thank goodness we had everything ready for him when he walked into the Great Hall early. It was one grand birthday party. Dasher did save some cake for Dancer—when he finally got there!"

Inside the Hall, Blitzen was directing several elves, who were hanging birthday greetings from the ceiling. Comet and Cupid were busy putting the final trimmings on an enormous birthday cake. Prancer and Mrs. Claus were just finishing setting up a huge table in the center. Everything sparkled! The long, wide banner hung from the ceiling across the entire room wished Dasher a "Happy Birthday" from everyone.

"Just how old, exactly, is Dasher?" I asked.

Vixen answered, for she was the one who kept up with the exact ages of all the Christmas Reindeer. "Let's see. Dasher started his Christmas service in the

Year of Our Lord 801. He was just a yearling buck back then, and his antlers had not fully grown out." Vixen looked at Donder. "If I remember correctly, I believe he still had a few fawn spots on him then."

Donder nodded. "Dasher was just a youngster when he came to the Pole."

Vixen continued, "Discounting space-time continuum, which adds 'years' to each of us every Christmas Eve, I calculate that Dasher is exactly 1,170 years old, North Pole years."

"What would that be in terms of mortal years?" I asked.

"Dasher would be about the age of a 12-year-old Reindeer, mortally speaking. That would be quite young, actually."

I leaned against the wall, amazed. This was too much for my mind.

Donder tried to help me out. "Immortality cannot be measured accurately by mortal standards," he explained. "Magic is forever! As long as there is laughter and happiness in one child's face, and as long as the winds of immortal Christmas circle the earth, we will live throughout time... and then some."

After giving me a moment to try to grasp that, Donder continued: "There is a set point in time, Lad, when each one of us will rejuvenate through our wisdom and age. In other words, at that point we will actually begin to grow younger! Then the process of Christmas immortality will begin again, and the cycle will just be repeated. Grandfather Blitzen is approaching his immortality set point, and in the span of several thousand years, he will start growing young again."

Donder advised me. "You don't have to understand it. Just believe in it."

"Yes," said Vixen. "What is important is the believing. It's like the tiny Child born so long ago in Bethlehem. His legacy and belief in Him have lasted for centuries. He guides the lives of the immortal Christmas Reindeer with His very being—through time and eternity. It is His love for us that bonds us together in our mission of caring and joy. It is the children who forever capture the magic and innocence of Christmas and gives it as a gift to all those young at heart—no matter their age."

"You're making perfect sense to me, Vixen," I assured her. And I felt the glow of Christmas fill my being from head to toe. I wanted to keep experiencing this love and happiness forever.

"You will, Lad," assured Donder, reading my thoughts. I asked him then if there was any way I could help other people feel this way too.

"Sure there is, Lad. Tell this story—tell these true Chronicles of the Christmas Reindeer. True believers will feel it and know it. And the magic will grow as more people choose to believe."

We were all respectfully quiet for a few moments after this discussion.

We continued to decorate as we waited for Dasher to return. A dozen or so elves were carrying packages into the Hall. They set them down on the big table. What gifts—all shapes and sizes! Donder added our present from Iceland to the pile.

Comet lit the candles, and as he did I was aware of a shrill, high-pitched sound that had been growing steadily in loudness for several minutes. Turning to Donder, who was grinning from ear to ear, I asked him what the sound was. It was then that I saw everyone running for the door to the Great Hall.

Dasher's Birthday and His Great Speed 193

Donder gripped me by the arm and said urgently, "Hurry, Lad, Dasher's coming! That's the sound you hear. It means Dasher is pushing wind molecules in front of him at an enormous rate of speed. If we're lucky, he might try to break the friction barrier. Vixen had mentioned earlier that because you're here, he might try to show off a little."

Donder, still holding onto my arm as we ran outside, said, "Lad, if Dasher does try to break the friction barrier, watch me and do exactly as I do, or else you'll have an earache for several days."

We hurried to join the crowd that had gathered just outside the door. Everyone was looking to the south. Vixen nudged my arm and pointed skyward, just over the horizon. Looking up, I saw that the sky had grown quite red and purple. The high-pitched whine not only grew louder—it became even more shrill, like a piercing whistle. The rushing wind also got stronger and began to blow some elves around. They grabbed at each other for added weight against its force. Blitzen even had several elves hanging to his massive antlers as he stood there, looking skyward.

Out to the south, I saw an orange glow just touching the horizon. It was continually glowing in brightness until it resembled a giant fireball accelerating at enormous speed.

"He's going for the barrier!" I heard someone shout. The orange fireball became even more brilliant. Then suddenly the orange glow disappeared and was instantly replaced by a blistering scarlet red color. I heard several voices loudly yell, "Take cover! He's going for the barrier! He's going to hit a magnitude 7!!!" There were several elves standing near me holding some type of electronic measuring device.

Donder quickly grabbed me, and with Vixen's help, dragged me to a rock wall just beside the Hall. Everyone, including Santa and Mrs. Claus, huddled down behind the wall. The noise was almost deafening! Even with my hands over my ears, I couldn't block it out. Donder poked me and pointed up. I looked, shielding my eyes. But what I saw is hard to describe.

The entire sky over the North Pole was brilliantly lit with sparkling colors. I saw a twinkling red fireball, and the glowing stardust trail that was shooting out behind the red fireball looked like the tail of a comet.

Donder quickly pulled some protective goggles over my head, down over my eyes. Looking closer at the fireball, I could just make out the shape of Dasher at the head of it. He was driving hard with his enormous antlers down in front of him. They gleamed like liquid gold, and the stardust from his antlers was showering the entire area with sparkling colors. It looked like millions of fireworks going off at the same time!

His legs were a blur, and a shimmering flame of blue was coming from each hoof. The brilliance was so great now, I had to shield my eyes even with the goggles on. It seemed as though I was looking straight into the sun. I realized that Dasher was going to pass far to the west of us. Donder explained later that Dasher had done this so he wouldn't cover the Pole with snow or blow any elves away.

As Dasher blistered by us, the wind became a shrill scream, and I saw what looked like the very atmosphere bulging outward. Then we heard a tremendous explosion—the sound of the friction barrier being broken.

Dasher's Birthday and His Great Speed

I reached out and quickly grabbed an elf that was sliding past me. He clung to me like glue, laughing his little head off. Donder had about six of them tucked under him for protection, as did the other Christmas Reindeer.

I watched as Dasher passed. Just behind him, a 300-foot wall of snow followed him like a tidal wave. The snow and ice had been dragged along in the vacuum of his speed. It passed by us with the roar of an ocean.

Dasher turned in a very wide arc and began to slow down. I saw the gleam and sparkle of his hooves begin to backtrack in motion. Dasher then started to climb to break his speed. He looked just like a shooting star. He shook the stardust from his antlers and created even more of a display.

"Well, he really did it this time," said Vixen, smiling. "Talk about showing off! I have never seen a display of speed to equal that before."

Dasher started to come in for his landing. He softly touched down some fifty yards away from the group. I heard and saw the snow sizzle as his hooves touched the cold snow. The clouds of steam rolled up around him, and for a moment, covered him completely.

Several elves ran toward him, holding what looked like fire extinguishers! They began to spray a white foam on his legs and hooves. The steam slowly subsided, and after the elves checked Dasher for stardust burn, he started walking toward us. We could feel the heat coming off him as he moved.

"That's from traveling so fast," explained Cupid. "It will take several days for his body to regain its normal temperature."

"The elves say he reached a magnitude of 7!" said Comet.

As we all stood around congratulating Dasher, Grandfather Blitzen cleared his throat and announced: "It's official, everyone. Dasher did achieve an acceleration of a magnitude 7.3 as he was going through the friction barrier. That's a North Pole record. No Christmas Reindeer has ever, by himself, with no emergency or special immortal help, gone that fast before!"

"I'm very proud of you, Dasher," congratulated Santa.

"Happy birthday, Dasher," shouted Cupid, pushing her way to the front of the group. And everyone started singing "Happy Birthday to You" as we trooped into the Great Hall of Toys.

Dasher, seeing all the presents and the big cake, began to cry with the excitement of it all. Elves started pushing him toward the cake. He wiped his eyes and was silent for a few moments. Then he said, "Thank you, everyone, for making this the greatest birthday of my life. You've all gone to so much trouble, just for me."

With this Dasher leaned over, and with a mighty puff of air, blew out all 1,170 candles! Everyone gave a great cheer and a round of applause. With Mrs. Claus' and Prancer's help, the cake was cut and pieces passed around.

Dasher had been guided to the chair of honor in the center of the room, and elves were bringing him birthday presents. It was grand.

Santa had given him a very handsome wood plaque, edged in gold. The inscription read: "Dasher (Hansrich), true and honest, born in the year of Christmas Magic, A.D. 800. Entered Christmas service for the

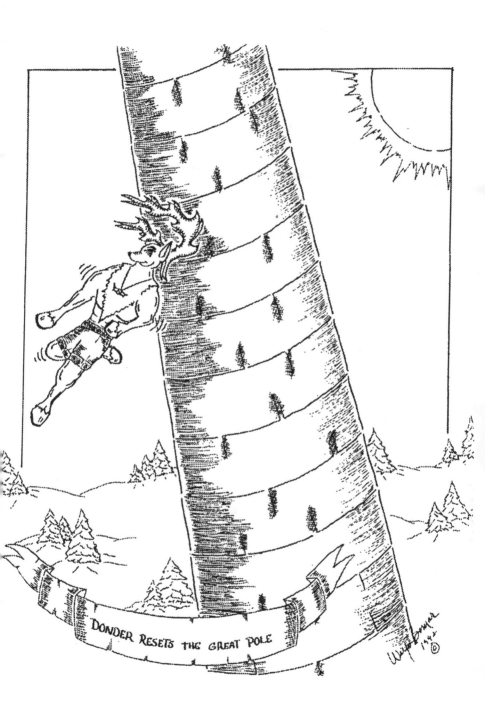

children of the world in the year A.D. 801. Birthplace: Husavik, Iceland. A noble and truthful Christmas Reindeer who has continued to serve the children of the world throughout time and eternity."

20

Dasher's Magical Story

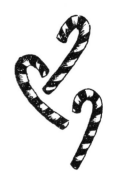

As everyone watched, Santa Claus hung the handsome plaque above the fireplace mantel. A great cheer went up throughout the Hall. We all started singing "For He's a Jolly Good Fellow!" Mrs. Claus gave Dasher a big kiss on the muzzle, and the rest of us patted him on the back.

Then one of the elves turned on the music, and Mrs. Claus asked Dasher if he would honor her with the first dance. We all watched, mesmerized, as they glided across the floor.

It was an enchanted night. After some six hours, the party started to wind down. The elves excused themselves, and after wishing Dasher a very happy birthday, they left the Great Hall for their beds. Soon there were only the Christmas Reindeer, Santa and Mrs. Claus, and myself left. We all sat around the big fireplace as Donder threw several more logs on.

It was Grandfather Blitzen who said, "I think now, Santa, would be a very good time to tell the story of how Dasher came to join our team."

"What a marvelous idea, Nicholas!" agreed Mrs. Claus. "Would you tell it?"

I quickly gathered some writing paper and looked around wildly for a writing utensil. Cupid and Vixen placed a small desk in front of me, and Donder left quickly to go retrieve my tape recorder. He returned just in time, as Santa began:

"Our beloved Dasher was the third-chosen among you. His christening name was Hansrich. It means "Truth and Honesty." Hansrich was born in the small fishing village of Husavik, Iceland, in the Year of Our Lord 800. Iceland, as you all know, is the land of the midnight sun.

"Blitzen and Donder had been in Christmas service for many years, before Dasher joined us. The great sleigh was becoming heavier and heavier, as our journey now covered so much more of the world. Blitzen and Donder required many days of rest after we returned home from our deliveries. So the three of us had been thinking very seriously that perhaps we needed another Christmas Reindeer to help us pull the load.

"This new Reindeer would have to be very special, we all agreed. He would have to love all children of all races in all countries—in all conditions.

"Each year as we traveled, we all searched for just that Reindeer. Our selection would have to be exactly correct. In 801, we set down in northern Iceland. We had been flying northeast across the top of the ice-covered country, and had planned to work our way south through Iceland, then on to other countries.

"I was quite concerned for Donder that Christmas Eve. He had come down with a bad cold and virus of some sort. As we traveled, I could feel his weakness as he struggled to keep up with Blitzen.

"I had already made up my mind to return home

and put Donder to bed, continuing the journey with just Blitzen. A hard pull for one Reindeer, but then again, Blitzen is no ordinary Reindeer." Santa patted Blitzen fondly on his shoulder.

"Iceland was a solitary country in those days, hardly settled at all, until the Norsemen came in around A.D. 850. Our stops in Iceland would not take very long, and then we could get Donder quickly back home. But just outside the small village of Husavik, Donder became very ill, collapsing in the cold snow. His breathing was very shallow, and as Blitzen and I rushed to his side, we were both fearful for him.

"Although Donder is immortal, a severe sickness of this nature could have left him weak for months. So we gathered him up and placed him in the sleigh, covering him with blankets. It had started to snow quite hard, and the runners of the great sleigh had frozen solid to the ice.

"Blitzen pulled and pushed mightily, but to no avail. The sleigh just simply wouldn't budge an inch. Donder, by this time, was wheezing badly, and we knew we had to get him back to the Pole where elf doctors could minister to him quickly!"

Santa paused for a moment to reach over and pat Donder's arm. Donder nodded his head and smiled as Santa continued: "I was terrified that he would get pneumonia, probably the most crippling illness that could befall a Christmas Reindeer.

"Blitzen and I strained for hours, but our efforts seemed in vain. The runners were stuck firm, and the bottom half of the sleigh was covered with snow. We even tried emptying the presents from the back compartment to lighten the load. But it was no use.

"We knew there was no help for miles, and so I

decided that Blitzen should carry Donder on his back, return to the Pole, and then come back for me. It was the only request he ever refused me! I'm so glad, as I would have frozen if he had done that.

"Donder was having an extremely hard time just breathing, and he had started to perspire heavily. That made the cold even more dangerous for him. So we tried to loosen the runners of the sleigh one more time — to no avail.

"Blitzen was beyond frightened now, as he was still a relatively young Reindeer, only 500 years old at that time. I tried not to show it, but Blitzen could see in my eyes that I thought all was lost. We huddled over Donder to protect him some from the driving snow — but my beard had frozen solid, and pieces of it were starting to break off, it was so cold!"

A feeling of anxiety almost overwhelmed me as I listened. It was so hard to imagine Santa in such a predicament.

"We thought of all that would perish if we gave up: Our Christmas Eve journeys would come to an end right there, in that snowstorm in Iceland. Blitzen cried out with despair, and it was a terrible sound. Yet I knew he was also imploring the Ancient of Ancients, the Christmas Immortals who forever keep watch over the Christmas Reindeer. His moans, from deep within his soul, spread farther out. They reverberated off every valley and canyon in that desolate, frozen country. With his head thrown back, Blitzen filled the skies with his cries for help.

"And then, from the white darkness of the lonely forest, a shadow suddenly appeared and moved slowly toward the sleigh — and us. I feared that wolves had been attracted to Blitzen's cries. I pulled Donder closer. But the dark shadow stopped just in front of us. It was Blitzen who rose to face the dark threat alone. He lowered his big antlers and stood erect, ready to give his life for us.

"Suddenly, the dark form before us spoke: 'I am Hansrich of Icelandia. Through a power unknown to me, with fierce and lordly voices, I have been summoned and guided here. Here I sense love and caring —the like of which I have never known before, except in the depth of my own heart for the children. I must help you—please, show me what I must do.'

"It was a magnificent reindeer that stood before us on his exceedingly muscular legs and spoke in the Icelandic tongue. He held his head high and proud, and we could tell that a great ancestry ran through his body. His soft eyes were filled with wonder as he gazed on us in our need.

"Blitzen quickly directed this young helper to Donder's empty harness. He seemed to know what to do. After hooking him into harness, Blitzen stood back. Hansrich lowered his big antlers, and with one powerful groan, leaped forward. There was a loud crack as one runner snapped loose from the hard ice. Again, and then again, Hansrich jumped forward with such strength that it jarred and shook the ground for many yards around us. The harness straps broke under his powerful pulling, and Blitzen quickly changed harnesses.

"Again, Hansrich strained with the weight of the sleigh. Then, with one final effort, he leaped forward and broke the other runner free as well! He walked forward several yards, pulling the great sleigh. Then he stood quietly, his head almost touching the snow, his sides heaving from exhaustion.

"Hansrich raised his head and whispered, 'O gracious Sinta Klauss... I now know why I was summoned here. You travel with the great Blitzen and the fine Donder. Your love and the miracle of your generosity is very dear to me, as you travel the night sky for the children's good. That is the most precious task in all the world. I, Hansrich, am here to assist you in any way I can, and for as long as you will need me.'"

Santa paused for a moment and looked deep into Dasher's eyes. Then he continued:

"I knew then, in my heart, that this magnificent Icelandic creature, Hansrich, was to become my third-chosen Christmas Reindeer. As I looked into his curious, wonder-filled eyes, I gently whispered, 'Journey with us, Hansrich, on our missions of love.'

"For a moment, Hansrich looked sad, and he answered, 'Would that I could, O Sinta Klauss, but I cannot fly like the great Blitzen and the fine Donder. Many tales I have heard of your magical journey. It is through the cries of the great Blitzen that I was sent to you. Could I but fly, O Sinta Klauss, gladly and with great love would I travel forever with you!'

"I looked at Blitzen, and knowing his heart as I do, I realized that he also knew what was to be Hansrich's destiny. Blitzen threw his mighty antlers back, and with a great cry toward the heavens, let out a sound that traveled beyond time. A twinkling of stardust appeared around Hansrich, and there in the snow he was bathed in the golden lights of the Beams of Immortality!

"The Ancient of Ancients had answered Hansrich's prayers! He had been granted his wish to travel with us to bring joy to the children he already loved so well.

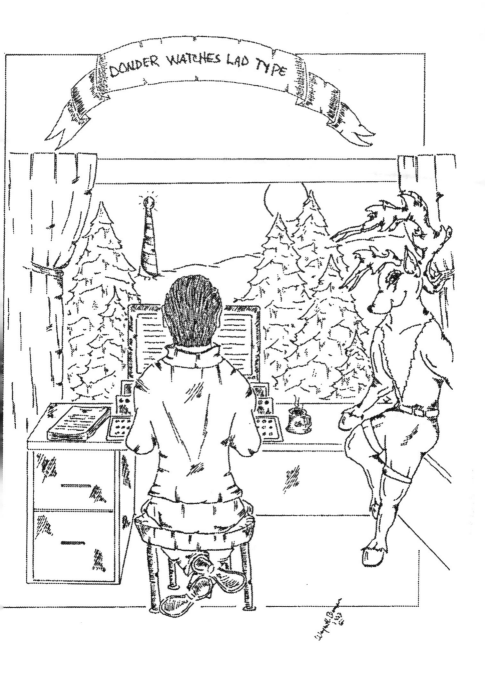

"Hansrich stood in the twinkling snow and glowed with the radiant light of immortal stardust. Blitzen slipped into the harness beside Hansrich and whispered, 'Do as I do, Hansrich of Iceland... learn the secrets of the stars and hear the laughter of the children of the world. Fill your heart with gladness and feel the wind-currents of a magical time. For it all lies before us!'

"I held tightly onto Donder as Blitzen took the lead. With Hansrich running beside him, we were by now silently skimming the crust of the snow. We started across an open field with frozen drifts that seemed a mile high. Hansrich obeyed, and soon I could feel the great sleigh lift a few feet into the air—only to bump softly down again!

"I could faintly hear Blitzen talking to Hansrich again. And then, with a great surge, we were suddenly airborne! We cleared the tall, snow-covered trees and sped on. Hansrich had some difficulty at first, but was absolutely jubilant at the feeling of freedom the open air gave him!

"Donder had regained consciousness and was watching through weak eyes as Hansrich and Blitzen turned toward the Great Star and home! With Hansrich's help, our speed increased and amazed us all. Donder finally raised his head slightly and whispered to me, 'He's quite a dasher, this Hansrich of Iceland.'

"At that time, Donder didn't know it, but he was giving Hansrich his Christmas name! For as we know, he is our Dasher, and no Reindeer could equal his speed—until Comet joined us nearly 700 years later! But that's another story.

"We landed at the Pole safely, with Blitzen once again taking the lead and setting us down gently outside the Great Hall. The elf doctors were standing by and they quickly bustled Donder off for treatment. When we knew he was safe and being ministered to, Blitzen, Dasher, and I again took to the skies to finish our Christmas Eve journey!

"Hansrich marveled at the magic of his first Christmas Eve flight. He behaved much like a child—as he really still was. He nearly wore us out! But, had it not been for Hansrich, there would have been no deliveries that Christmas Eve—and possibly never again."

Santa paused silently for a moment.

"When we returned, Hansrich went to see the recovering Donder, first thing. It was almost as if they had already become brothers. Donder became his teacher, his comrade, his true friend. And so 'Dasher' has been with us ever since. He was truly destined to become a Christmas Reindeer, and we all love him very, very much!"

Dasher had listened silently to the whole of Santa's story. His face showed his great emotion, but he then also stood up and told us: "There is no way I can fully express my love for all of you. You're my family."

Many hugs were passed around. Then Blitzen took his mug of punch and proposed a toast: "To Hansrich, the third-chosen of the Christmas Reindeer, aye! We drink this birthday toast to you, on your day. You have brought much happiness to the children of the world, and have served faithfully, in truth and honesty, through many immortal years. We salute you, Hansrich of Icelandia!"

There was not much anyone could say or do after that wonderful ending to the evening. Donder and I helped Dasher load up his birthday presents, and then said good-night and went out. We walked back to Donder's house.

Donder turned to me quietly and said, "Now that you are telling our stories, everyone will know who Dasher really is and all that he has done for the children of the world."

I pulled back the curtain in my room and looked across the snow. I could just see Dasher's house from my window—and inside I saw Dasher sitting at his writing table. I smiled and lay down. I drifted off to sleep and dreamed of riding with Dasher across the night into a twinkling sunset.

21

A Get-Together at Cupid's

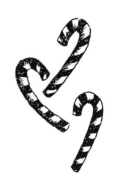

The next morning, Donder and I hustled off to the toy factory to see if we could help with anything. We wandered around Dasher's department, doing this and that. I noticed that Donder had stopped to talk with Dasher about a get-together at Cupid's house later that evening.

After a brief visit to Comet's department, Donder and I wandered around the Pole. Donder explained some of the sights I was seeing, which I eagerly wrote down in the ever-present notepad I held. I will try to describe some of those wonders here.

There were the ice falls in many splendid colors... Prancer's pinnacles of ice that overlooked the Great North Sea... the much-kept secret entrance to the North Pole... Grandfather Blitzen's ice cove, where he kept his small sailboat (he sometimes went out into the ice flows to call to his beloved whales)...

Donder even showed me where the mysterious "Snow Witzels" lived. They were curious, docile creatures that lived far beneath the ice packs of the Pole. Donder explained to me that the "Witzels" had been driven almost to extinction. They had wandered far to the North, where Santa Claus had given them sanctuary forever! Donder chuckled and told me that you have to look very close to see a Snow Witzel. He and the other Reindeer would often go in search of the creatures in many a fun-filled sleigh ride down the ice mountains.

I said I would love to see one. Donder smiled and said, "In due time, Lad... in due time. They are very shy, and terrified of people. But they know you're here."

"How do you know?" I asked, astonished.

He stopped and whispered to me, "Because they have been following us for the last 30 minutes!"

I turned around, but saw nothing—just drifts of snow and ice. "Where are they?" I asked.

"Believe me, Lad, they're here. You'll see them another time, as well as other creatures you'll find absolutely amazing."

"What other creatures, Donder?"

"Over the centuries, Lad," he explained, "many species have been hunted, and their race almost destroyed. Many came here, to the great ice flats of the North Pole, to be under the protection of the good Santa Claus. Santa gave them refuge and loved them. He vowed to protect all who came. Never again will they be hunted and destroyed!"

"How wonderful!" I exclaimed.

"Yes, without the love of Santa Claus, they might have perished from the earth forever."

We started walking back, and went over to see Vixen in the mailroom. Then we stopped by the Great Hall to chat with Dancer, Prancer, and Cupid. It seemed that Donder had set everything up for the evening's gathering at Cupid's. I did so look forward to these times, as each story gave me insight into the history—and the heart—of one of the Christmas Reindeer.

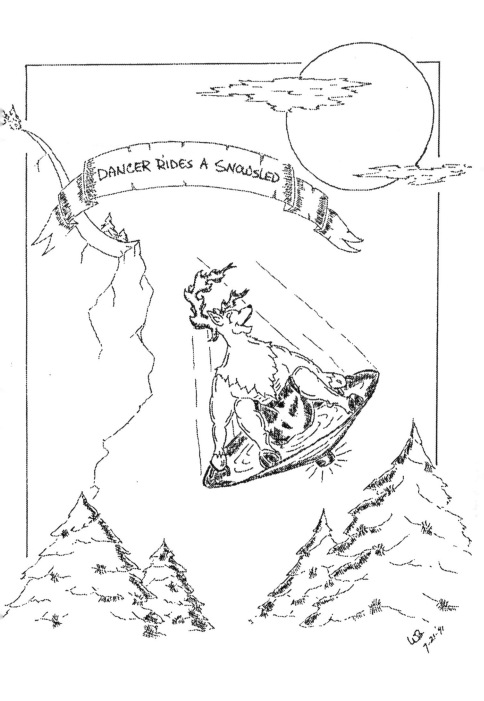

Tonight would be very special, as Grandfather Blitzen and Donder had graciously agreed to tell the story of how Comet had joined them on their journeys. I gathered together my tape recorder, paper, and pens.

Donder had told me a bit about Cupid's house. She was a very modern Reindeer—the only one who slept in a water bed and had shiny, white shag carpet throughout her home. She had bean-bag chairs around a circular fireplace in the middle of her living room, he said. I couldn't wait to see it!

We went to get dressed for the evening, and I found that we had special gifts waiting on our beds: beautiful black sweaters with glittery silver stitching in the form of lightning bolts down the arms. On the front were portraits of Comet with the words: "Vasha —A.D. 951. May the wind be at your back, your course clear, your path truthful."

"They're from Cupid and Vixen," Donder explained.

"Wow!" I exclaimed as I pulled mine on.

"I will tell you ahead of time that Comet comes from the northernmost part of Finland, and that his name means 'Brother of the Wind.'"

My eyes bulged. This was going to be quite an evening. Blitzen was bringing his chip wafers, and I was told Mrs. Claus had baked for us her world-famous "Rocky Road North Pole Pie."

I had one more question for Donder: "Exactly how fast can Comet run?"

"No one knows for certain," he said. "Just as none of us had ever seen Dasher fly that fast before yesterday. I don't think even Comet knows for sure his own limits. I will tell you this, Lad. Comet can move out when he needs to, but I don't think he has ever reached his true potential yet—his top speed."

A Get-Together at Cupid's

I thought about that all the way over to Cupid's house.

"Come in, come in," she greeted us at the door. Everyone else except for Comet was already there. They were all wearing sweaters identical to the "Comet" sweaters we had been given by Cupid and Vixen.

Donder had certainly been right about Cupid's house being modern—from the shag carpet to the frosty, white walls. Everyone looked quite comfortable in the bean-bag chairs, too. But most unusual was the way her ceiling opened up to the sky. She had a beautiful curved skylight that allowed you to look up and see the Great Star shining down! It was absolutely breathtaking.

The light beams made the stardust twinkle in the antlers of each Reindeer. For the first time I noticed that Santa's beard and Mrs. Claus' hair were faintly sparkling with stardust. As though understanding my sudden discovery, Cupid handed me a mirror and told me to look at my own hair. I had to catch my breath! My hair, too, was shimmering with tiny flecks of stardust!

"My hair! Has it always been like that?" I asked, astonished.

Grandfather Blitzen smiled warmly. "Aye, Lad! That it has—ever since you came. You just couldn't see it before. It's the magic, of course."

"Isn't this exciting!" bubbled Cupid, as she led us to chairs beside Blitzen and Dasher. Both of them were to be the storytellers tonight.

We awaited the arrival of Comet at 7:00—just a few minutes to go. Prancer put more logs on the fire, and Mrs. Claus began serving the punch, which was flavored with cinnamon. After what seemed forever, there was a knock on the door. Cupid tiptoed over to open it.

There outside stood a smiling Comet. His mouth dropped immediately, however, when he saw us all sitting there wearing the identical sweaters with his portrait on them!

Vixen came forward, and with Cupid's help, pushed him into the living room and placed him in a chair just opposite Santa, Dasher, and Blitzen. Comet was speechless. He just sat there, stunned.

Santa burst out laughing. "This is a first, if I say so myself! I've never seen Comet so quiet before!"

That broke the ice, and everyone started talking and laughing at the same time. Mrs. Claus came up and gave Comet a big hug and a kiss on the muzzle. Comet stared at her, puzzled. She whispered in his ear, "Tonight's your night, Dear. It's just for *you*."

I was amazed at Comet's reaction. That proud, speedy Christmas Reindeer looked so innocent and vulnerable.

I knew that soon Comet's story would be told. I got ready to start writing, while Santa tamped his pipe out. Cupid and Vixen sat down beside Comet and were holding his hooves in theirs.

Vixen whispered, "It's a beautiful story, Vasha. Now the world will be told of the love you have given the children for so many years."

I was on the edge of my seat as Santa began:

"It was in the Year of Our Lord 885. By now I had my beloved Reindeer, Blitzen, Donder, Dancer, and Prancer, who made up the Christmas team. The tales about us had indeed spread throughout the world. Each year's flight was even more beautiful than the last. There were always more children who needed toys and gifts, as the world's population had grown even larger.

"Blitzen, Donder, Dasher, and I discussed the possibility of finding yet another Reindeer to help pull the enormous load. We decided that we would not rush into anything. We would wait, as we had done before, and let the magic guide us. Little did we know that the wonderful Christmas magic was already at work!"

He relit his pipe and continued: "He was born in the year 884 in a very small village called Inari, in the far North of Finland, many miles above the Arctic Circle. You might have called him the runt of the litter, he was so tiny when he was born.

"His mother named him 'Vasha,' which in Finnish means 'Brother of the Wind.' He had bright, curious eyes, very large and brown. The most extraordinary thing about him, however, was the *natural symbol of a lightning bolt* that appeared in his antlers when he was old enough to grow them. He was not frightened of much, as he wandered quite close to humans, even from his early days.

"Vasha discovered very early in his young life that he could run. He was faster than the wind! Vasha could quite easily outdistance any of the other animals that inhabited the forest. After all, there *was* that symbol of the lightning bolt in his antlers.

"Vasha lingered near the children of the small village, and soon he became a devoted friend of all the children. He could detect, or hear, the cry of a small child for many miles, wondering at his own amazing ability. It was something he just couldn't ignore.

"He would often stand at the edge of the deep woods until he was sure a lost child had been found.

Many a child he carried to safety on his back after a misadventure or injury. The children soon learned that they had only to call to Vasha, and he would hear them and soon find them.

"Yet, in his heart, Vasha had a deep longing. What it was he wished for, he didn't know. Still, this inner sadness remained and grew in intensity. Vasha somehow felt the need in his soul *to help all the children of the world.*

"Often he would run toward the North, covering many miles in a short time, and marvel at how he could accomplish this. Then Vasha would stand on the lonely ice and search the skies until he found the Great Star of the North. He would stand and cry for many hours, all alone, not knowing why.

"With his family, he sat and listened long into the dark nights to the stories that were told of the good Sinta Klauss and his magical Christmas Reindeer. He learned how they traveled the world every Christmas and brought joy and happiness to those who believed in the spirit and the magic of Christmas.

"Often he would travel the many miles to the edge of the ice, far to the North. There, he would stand and wait, searching the heavens for the stardust trail that the magical Christmas Reindeer leave behind them as they fly the wind-currents of Christmastime.

"Several times, he thought he saw the stardust trail. Vasha would run like the wind, following the twinkles of magic in the sky, in hopes of catching them.

"Vasha would journey for many miles like this, running until he thought he would collapse with exhaustion. 'So near,' he would think, 'but why can't I catch them? I want to be with them!' he would cry to the wind.

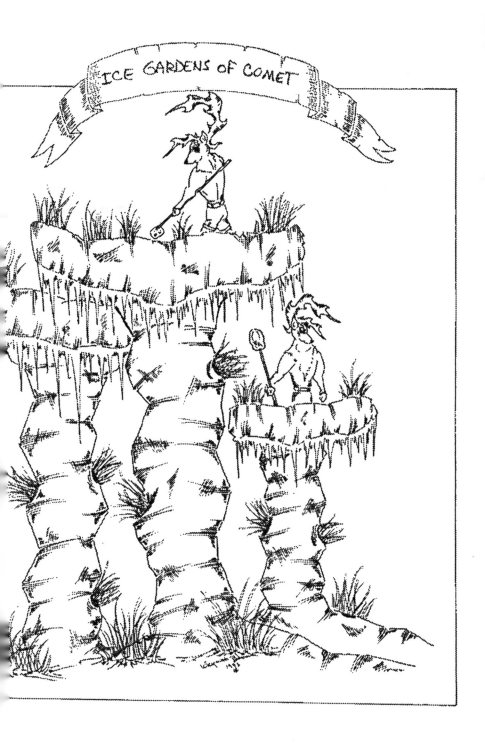

"'I can help,' he would think. As Vasha would watch the stardust trails faintly disappear below the horizon, he would turn slowly and sadly to his village. Vasha wrote many letters to us, expressing his desire and longing to journey with us, and to spread love to the children, using his own unique gifts."

As Blitzen spoke these words, he began to reach into his pocket. I felt a stirring of suspense and magic in the very air of Cupid's living room as I waited for the next revelation about Vasha, our very own Comet, Brother of the Wind.

22

Comet: Brother of the Wind

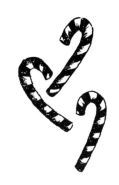

Grandfather Blitzen paused for a moment as he recalled for us the story of Comet. Then he pulled from his pocket many letters, now faded in color due to great age. He handed these to me and said, "Please read the top letter, Lad. It was the last one written by Vasha to us before he joined our North Pole family."

I carefully opened the yellowed envelope that had been sent to Grandfather Blitzen hundreds of years ago by Comet. It read: "Dear Sinta Klauss and Wonderful Reindeer of Christmas: It is Vasha who writes to you again. If in some way I might be of service to you, you have but to say the word.

"I am writing this letter on behalf of a small child who lies very ill. She has brought me great happiness and joy through her smiles as she rides with me through our snowy woods. Her laughter used to fill the lonely forest. Now she is very sick and can only lie in her bed. She is very weak now, and this is why I am writing to you.

"Little Elainya, for that is her name, has told me many wonderful stories about the magical Reindeer as only a child can tell. Elainya sees you through the eyes of child-magic. Her only wish is to touch the muzzle of the great Blitzen and let him know that she loves him very much.

"Elainya has shown me letters that the kind Blitzen has written to her. His devoted love for all children fills each letter she has received. If only you knew what joy those letters have brought to her!

"Such happiness I have never seen on the face of a child. Yet, some nights ago, in her fever, she reached out to me and touched my face and whispered, 'How I love you, Grandfather Blitzen.' For a moment, she thought I was the magical Blitzen!

"At that instant, I was privileged to feel as *you* must feel when a child reaches out to you in love and hope. As Elainya became unconscious from her fever, I ran toward the North, to stand upon the ice ridge, and there I cried for Elainya. She must not leave us, Grandfather. *You must come.* It will save little Elainya, I know that it will.

"Through your magic and great love, you can save Elainya. I beg of you, Grandfather, please come and allow her to but touch you and gaze in your eyes. I know this will cure her. She is so tiny, yet so filled with love. Please..."

The letter was signed simply: "Vasha, of Finland, your servant always." I looked at Comet, who still had his head bowed slightly. Vixen and Cupid were holding Comet about his shoulders now, very tightly. Comet's antlers were quivering ever so slightly, and I know that he was remembering those precious moments of so long ago.

Grandfather Blitzen wiped his eyes, and, looking at Dasher, nodded his antlers. Dasher then picked up the story where Blitzen had left off: "Of course, after reading the letter from Vasha, there was no question that Grandfather would go see little Elainya. He simply had to do whatever he could for this child, who loved him so much. I accompanied Grandfather on this journey, and we arrived in the small village of Inari a day later.

"That night, through the magic of love and belief, Grandfather stood beside little Elainya's bed. The child—upon seeing Blitzen the great Christmas Reindeer standing there, stardust twinkling in his massive antlers—threw her tiny, wasted arms around his neck. She told him of her love for him and the other magical Reindeer, and how she would love him forever.

"She begged Grandfather to take her with him, as she was so very tired of lying in her bed, unable to run and play or do anything. 'I know you can help me heal, Grandfather,' she said simply.

"I listened through the open window as little Elainya told Grandfather of how she used to have such fun. She told of her special friend Vasha, who always came to see her, and how she used to ride with him through the forest.

"Elainya prattled on as a child would talk. And, as Grandfather knelt beside the little girl, he could sense what was causing her illness! She finally relaxed her hold from around his neck, and slowly sank back into her bed.

"Blitzen, gently shaking his antlers, covered little Elainya with twinkling stardust to relieve her pain awhile.

"Once we had left her home, Grandfather sadly told me that, as things were, the child would not live through the night. But a medicine *did* exist that could possibly cure her. Shaking his head, he lamented,

'There's not enough time, Dasher... not enough time. The stardust I have covered her with will relieve her pain only for a short while. The fever again will come, and I fear she is not strong enough now to withstand it.'

"I'll never forget what Grandfather told me then as we stood outside the child's house in the softly falling snow. He said that even I, with my great speed, might not be swift enough to go for the medicine and back again, so sick was little Elainya.

"Grandfather told me that this medicine of powerful curing abilities did exist, far to the West in a small group of islands inhabited by the Fairies of Crystalix. They are the makers of white magic. The fairies, Grandfather said, would gladly give of the medicine that might save little Elainya. But, the journey was very long, and there was so little time. Would I try? he asked. There was no hesitation as I accepted this task.

"He described to me the route I must fly. I was not to stop for anything, and every second was precious. I had just turned to leave when he held up his arm and said, 'WAIT! Dasher, there might be another way. Vasha, come here quickly!'

"I turned and saw a young reindeer bound from the edge of the dark woods. Grandfather had known all of the time that young Vasha stood quietly there listening and watching what was happening to his friend Elainya.

"Vasha slid to a stop in front of Blitzen and bowed low before him. Grandfather laid his arm on Vasha's shoulder and quietly whispered, 'It is the love of a child that has brought us here. It is your love, Vasha, that might save her. Your great speed will become even greater because of your love. You know the route you must take. The Fairies of Crystalix will know I have sent you. Fly, Vasha, FLY!'"

Dasher smiled through his tears of remembrance and said, "Grandfather motioned for me to follow Vasha, lest something befall him on his urgent mission. Quickly I turned to go after him, but he was already gone in a swirl of stardust. Blitzen had bestowed upon Vasha the gift of flight for this important task. I followed his stardust trail and found where he had lifted himself up into the cold wind-currents of the night sky.

"Such speed I had never seen before! Even I could not catch him. I knew and understood how he was able to do this. It was deep, sincere love that carried Vasha through the darkness with hope in his heart.

"I sensed his approach to the islands of Crystalix, and again sensed his takeoff from the islands. I could feel his closeness as I searched the dark sky for sight of him.

"Finally, just over the horizon, I caught a glimpse of him. I was immediately frightened for him. Vasha had not yet learned how to use the protected aura of Christmas magic that surrounds each of us and keeps the immense heat of fast flight from burning us up. Vasha had not slowed down at all, but continued to gain momentum.

"The friction from his great speed was devastating! I could feel the heat coming off him from miles away. I was afraid he would be burned up! I began to will with all my heart that my magic aura would surround and safely protect him for the remainder of his journey. This was miraculously granted, and Vasha passed me in a blur of white, brilliant light.

"I had to travel slowly now, for without my magic

aura to surround me, I would surely fall to the ground below, I was so weak. I could only hope that Vasha, with his great speed, would make it back in time for Blitzen to give little Elainya the medicine.

"Finally, I arrived back in Inari. Standing beside the window of the little girl's room was Vasha, his head down and his body limp. Yet his only concern was for Elainya.

"As I stood there beside him, he whispered, 'Thank you... for what you gave me. Without your gift I could not have made it.'

"It was just then that we both heard the voice of Elainya. She was telling Grandfather Blitzen how much better she felt, and that she knew he could make her well again. 'Aye, 'twas not I,' he said, 'but your friend Vasha who carried the miracle to you, for he loves you so very much.'

"The child reached out to Vasha, and as he stepped closer, she threw her arms around his neck crying, 'O Vasha, how can I ever thank you? You have given me back my life!'

"As Vasha bent down, we could see that his antlers had started to melt during the flight, and he had singed fur due to the great speed he had attained. For many long minutes, we stood and gazed upon him and the child.

"Then Grandfather sensed that he and I were having the same thoughts. He said aloud, 'Vasha, you have proved your faith and love for children in what you have done tonight. You would have gladly given your life for this child. Such love is the miracle above all things on this earth. Journey with us now, Vasha, as Christmas Reindeer together—and know the love and joy of children forever!'

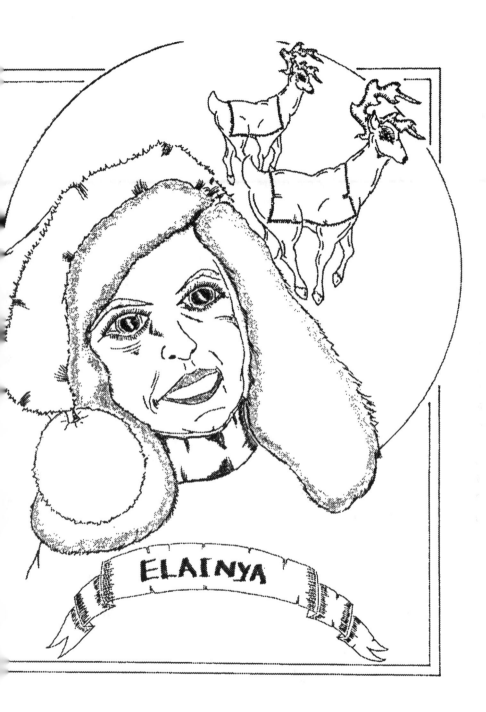

"Vasha turned to Grandfather, his eyes wide with wonder. 'It is what I have longed for all my life,' he cried. And little Elainya squealed with joy, for she understood the great gift that was being given to her friend Vasha. He would be a Christmas Reindeer throughout time and eternity!

"Grandfather put his arm on Vasha's shoulder and whispered, 'She'll be well again, now, Vasha. Never fear. You will see her again soon.'

"After we had said our final good-byes, Vasha left with us. We leaped into the night sky and returned home to the North Pole. Ever since that night, Vasha has been one of us. He has loved and served the children of the world faithfully and devotedly! And that is the story of our marvelous friend, Comet, for all the world to know."

I was so glad the tape recorder was on, for I couldn't have written a word, I was so filled with deep feeling. Santa then spoke up clearly, "Little Elainya did get well. She grew into a fine, beautiful woman, and married. She had three strong sons and two lovely daughters. Eventually, she told the story of Vasha to her children, and they in turn have told it to theirs. The story has never been forgotten.

"Today, there stands a monument to Vasha in the small town of Inari, set there by Elainya's children. It honors what he did that night for a small, sick child. The last line reads simply: 'I love you, Vasha.' It was Elainya's wish that it should speak to generations of his great honor and courage—and be a beacon of hope to those who doubt or are weak. It was his love that made it all possible."

Grandfather Blitzen had arisen and was now standing beside Comet. "There is another strand to this story," he said. "Over the mantel in Comet's home is an oil portrait of a little girl with golden hair. She holds a white flower in her hands, and she smiles the smile of an angel. It is, of course, a portrait of Elainya. He is able to see this likeness of her every morning upon rising, and every night before lying down.

"Vasha has many special children, but little Elainya is the most special of all. I know that he still thinks of her often, and of how much he loves her."

Vixen had gotten up and disappeared into Cupid's bedroom for a moment. She returned holding a special sweater that she held out to Comet. On the front of it was a portrait of a little girl with golden hair smiling the smile of an angel. It was Elainya.

Comet looked at the sweater for a long minute, then stood up and put it on over his shirt. He looked around at all of us and said with feeling, "I love you all so much. I will treasure this evening, this wonderful sweater, and the precious memories of Elainya." At that his voice broke and he could say no more.

Cupid stood on the tips of her hooves to reach him and hug him tightly. Mrs. Claus was crying as she did the same. "Such a beautiful story, Comet, 'Brother of the Wind'! We are so proud of you!"

Later, after we returned to Donder's house, I knew I had to stay up and work further on the book. I wrote until dawn, when, looking out the window, I saw Comet come out of his house on his way to work. He turned and looked at me and smiled. He was wearing his new sweater.

He slowly turned and walked down the hill through the gently falling snow, stardust sparkling in his antlers.

23

Dancer and Prancer: A Tale of Great Reindeer

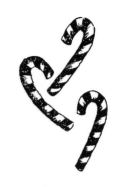

As I write these *Chronicles of the Christmas Reindeer*, I realize that there are sometimes no words for what I am trying to describe. These wonderful Reindeer have become my family. And they all know how much I love them.

And so I try to show that love in the way I am telling their stories. There is one more story to tell—a history of a call to serve the children of the world. It is that of Dancer and Prancer, two great Christmas Reindeer!

But now I must hurry. Donder and I are on our way to Prancer's house to join the others.

The weather had turned quite cold. The snow was falling thick and fast, so that I could barely make out the big Christmas tree in the center of the Reindeer compound. After we had put on our heavy topcoats and wrapped scarves around our necks, Donder put our contribution to the dinner tonight into a brown woolen bag and said, "Ready, Lad?"

Halfway across the compound, we were joined by Dasher and Vixen, also bundled up snugly. When we got to Prancer's door I was delighted that his doorbell was a set of chimes that played "Silent Night"! "Welcome to my home," he said warmly to us all.

We scurried inside and found the others already there. I had a good feeling that this night too would be very special.

Prancer's Christmas tree was a brilliant green with red ribbons and little wooden shoes all over it—reflecting his Dutch heritage. Each of the wooden shoes was filled with tiny packages in bright Christmas paper!

After everyone had filled plates with the wonderful treats, and taken mugs of hot chocolate, we all sat comfortably around the fire.

Grandfather Blitzen cleared his throat and said, "Neeki, Meirkos..." Dancer and Prancer started, looked quickly at Blitzen, then at me. I had never heard their christening names before!

The magical story of Dancer and Prancer was about to begin. Blitzen said, "Lad, be ready to write, for tonight you will hear how Neeki and Meirkos also became Christmas Reindeer. They joined us as a pair—the only two to have done so. They are inseparable, and have been for nearly 1,150 years.

"Neeki and Meirkos were born in the Year of Our Lord 838, in the small village of Medemblik, in the Netherlands. They were and are first cousins. Their parents all knew that they were destined for something wonderful, from the day they were born.

"Dancer was named 'Neeki' on a cold, clear day in 838. His name in Dutch means 'Magical Laughter.' Prancer, born on the same day, was named 'Meirkos,' or 'Children's Keeper' in Dutch.

"Even as they took their first wobbly steps, they

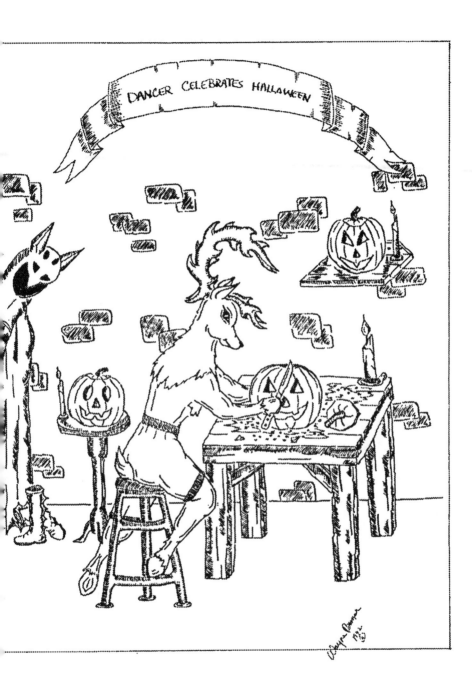

were always together. There was never such a pair as Neeki and Meirkos! And wherever they went, there were children. Neeki would make children laugh at his antics, and Meirkos would always be there if they needed help."

Donder interrupted Blitzen at this point to say, "The day they were born, Grandfather Blitzen announced their birth to all of us. He said that these two were born for the children, and that we must watch them grow, for the children's sake."

Vixen added, "It was a miracle, what happened on that special day in Medemblik. You," she said, looking at Dancer and Prancer, "are both here because of it. It was because the children loved you so very much."

Then Blitzen continued: "As Neeki and Meirkos grew, they continued to watch over the young ones of the village. They would ice skate with the children on frozen, ice-twinkling canals. They sometimes pulled them in sleds for hours at a time! It was a wonderful growing-up time.

"And while they were both young, they began to hear strange voices inside their heads. As they grew older, the whispers became more distinct. The voices said, over and over again, 'Believe in us, believe in the magic, believe in the children...'

"They both wondered at this, and would talk to each other about what they had heard and what it all meant. Yet they continued to be happy and content with their lives. They continued to play with and help the village children. And when they were around, the people of Medemblik always knew their children were safe.

"Every Christmas Eve, they would stand with the

children and search the skies with them for any sign of the good Sinta Klauss and his magical Christmas Reindeer.

"In the village of Medemblik lived a very old and wise man, who had proclaimed for many years that two of their own would be chosen to bring happiness to their children and to the children of the world. Neeki and Meirkos would sit with the children and listen to this old man tell stories of Sinta Klauss and the wonderful flying Reindeer.

"On one special Christmas Eve, the old man came to stand beside Neeki and Meirkos as they searched the skies. Standing with one arm on each of them, he whispered, 'Of all the villagers, you are the special ones.' On that night, the faint twinkling of stardust first appeared in their antlers.

"What Neeki and Meirkos didn't know was that the children had written hundreds of letters asking if Neeki and Meirkos could be granted the gift to journey with us as Christmas Reindeer, pulling the great sleigh of miracles. These children never asked anything for themselves—it was always this request for the two of you," Blitzen said, looking at the Reindeer of honor.

"They were the ones who wanted you to be called to live forever as immortal Christmas Reindeer, to share the joy and laughter with all the world. Not a day went by that we didn't get at least one letter.

"And then, in early spring, the miracle Vixen spoke of... happened.

"It was the spring of 839, and the previous winter had brought much snow to the village. Each year in Medemblik, the people celebrated the post-Christmas season with a huge Christmas picnic. Everyone in the village looked forward to this annual event on a snow meadow at the outskirts of the village.

"Among those at this picnic were Neeki and Meirkos. The meadow was beautiful that day with the huge ice mountain looming over it, still covered with heavy snow.

"The children scampered here and there, squealing with laughter at Neeki's antics. Then—suddenly, Neeki stopped stone-cold. Meirkos, too, had sensed the danger, like a warning from deep within.

"They had both come to trust these inner thoughts, because of the voices which still spoke to them. As they suddenly stopped the play and began looking for the danger area, the children looked at them, puzzled.

"Neeki and Meirkos looked this way and that, but they could see nothing unusual. Then Neeki realized what it was, and shouted that dreaded word: 'AVALANCHE!' Both of them turned to face the mountain that reared up before them. The keen hearing of these two picked up the distant sound of faint, rolling thunder—it was really the sound of ice cracking from deep within the mountain!"

Donder picked up the story at this point:

"Back at the North Pole, we all realized that these children and villagers were in great danger—at the very moment that Neeki and Meirkos knew it too. Blitzen, Dasher, and I were already in our traces. Santa bounded from his house and leaped into the sleigh. With a tremendous burst of energy, we were airborne and flying fast toward Medemblik. We flew like the wind, searching for air-currents that would enable us to travel faster. We were frantic, fearful we could not reach them in time.

"In our minds, we saw the top of the ice mountain breaking loose and starting to hurtle snow and ice onto the children far below. To lighten our load, Santa dumped all excess weight out of the sleigh—and we increased our speed even more.

"In our minds we saw Neeki and Meirkos warning the people, and children climbing on the reindeer's backs to try to escape to safety. At that very moment we envisioned ice and snow plummeting rapidly down the side of the mountain."

Donder looked at Blitzen and added, "It was as we realized there was no way we could make it, that Grandfather brought the great sleigh to a complete, sudden stop. It was his will alone that held us aloft in midair. Dasher and I realized at once what he intended to do. We looked at each other in disbelief. It seemed impossible!

"Dasher and I could sense Grandfather's inner voice calling to Neeki and Meirkos so far away, telling them again and again, 'Believe in us, believe in the magic, *believe in the children!*'

"And—well—a miracle is the only word to describe what happened. From outside Medemblik, Neeki and Meirkos heard Grandfather calling to them. Feeling his inner strength and his faith pouring into them, they received the great gift of flight. They soon found themselves soaring over the snow-covered meadow, scooping children up and flying them to safety.

"Swiftly they worked, as they listened, oh so carefully, to Grandfather's instructions. They didn't stop to wonder at the magic, they just trusted it—while snow and ice continued to thunder down the mountain.

"They were literally flying against time to save the children. The villagers who had reached safety by now marveled at the great clouds of stardust coming from Neeki and Meirkos! Great trees were snapped in two as the heavy ice flattened the ground and blistered onward, toward a small group of children who had not yet reached safety.

"Neeki and Meirkos turned back toward this group. With an awful, desperate scream of anguish and determination, they both launched themselves straight at the high-moving wall of ice and snow that—in an eyeblink—would have covered the children.

"At that moment, that precise instant, our own magical Christmas auras poured into Neeki and Meirkos. As they collided with the solid wall of ice and snow, we heard them hit head-on with a tremendous impact. The stardust explosion was seen for miles.

"Of course, we hoped for the best, but feared the worst.

"We then sensed, happily and miraculously, that the wall of snow and ice had parted when Neeki and Meirkos had collided with it. It had hurtled past the children, never touching a one of them!

Grandfather Blitzen picked up the story again: "And so, on that fateful day, the children—738 of them—were saved by the courage of Neeki and Meirkos. However, at the impact, Neeki and Meirkos' magic auras had been broken. We instantly lost our contact with them.

"We continued on our journey to Medemblik to rejoice at this victory, and to help carry the exhausted people back home. When we arrived in Medemblik we looked around for Neeki and Meirkos. Where were they, after their great feat?

"Donder found Neeki, just inches from Meirkos. We pulled them from the snow, limp and lifeless. Santa carried them in his strong arms and laid them gently down beside the great sleigh. The stardust still twinkled in their antlers, but since they were still but mortal reindeer, we feared the Ancients had called them home.

"Santa sat in the snow and cradled their heads in his lap and cried. The children clung to him and to the limp forms of Neeki and Meirkos. These two had given everything they had to give—themselves! But then, like the whisper of wind on a clear, starlit night, or the sound of a leaf falling, we heard soft voices coming from the mountains—softly at first, but then growing in intensity.

'For the love of but one child is the most powerful force imaginable. As the love of all children will remain forever, so shall these two remain forever. O Nicholas, it is into your keeping that we place these two gentle creatures of love. The children's hopes and dreams have been answered this day, and through the love of these very same children, Neeki and Meirkos shall remain forever as immortal Christmas Reindeer!'

"Santa had gotten up and was standing just behind Neeki and Meirkos, his arms raised to the mountains.

"Just then we heard a soft whimper of life! It came from Neeki! All was still as we watched their lifeless forms. Then Meirkos suddenly gulped in a lungful of air, his snow-covered body twitching with life. Neeki opened his dazed eyes and very gently reached for Meirkos, who lay beside him. Meirkos opened his eyes slowly and reached for Neeki. Their eyes grew wide with wonder as they looked upon the good Santa Claus. All of the children who remained with us cried with joy and relief.

"The tired reindeer struggled weakly to their feet, and stood facing us, heads bowed. They said, 'Bless you for saving the children.' Santa smiled and knelt down in front of them, placing his big hands on their shoulders, and said, ''Twas not we who saved the children. 'Twas their faith and love for both of you that saved them.' Then, with a wave of his arm, he faced the people still present and said, 'Look upon them, faithful people of Medemblik! For this day, now and forever, throughout time, these reindeer of your blessed village shall be true Christmas Reindeer!'

"Great shouts and cheering rang out through the crowd. The children were jubilant. Their beloved Neeki and Meirkos would journey throughout time with the good Sinta Klauss—as immortal Christmas Reindeer. The celebrations of this great day were to last a very long time.

"At the end of the day, Santa and I led Neeki and Meirkos to the great sleigh. They stood trembling with happiness as we helped them into harness. The villagers watched as we jumped into the night sky—to take Neeki and Meirkos home."

Then Santa said, "Each year now, Lad, as you know, the small village of Medemblik honors Neeki and Meirkos—Dancer and Prancer, as their Christmas names now are—with the 'Festival of the Reindeer.' They are my fourth- and fifth-chosen Reindeer, and I love them both so very much! They will never be forgotten for what they did that day, and for the great gift that was given to them."

Donder turned to me in the great emotion that we all felt, and reminded me, "Put it down, Lad. Just as we have told it. I'll be nearby tonight as you work, should you need me."

And so, after we returned to Donder's house, I typed through the night and into the next day. And as I finished the Chronicle of Dancer and Prancer, I looked out and saw them walking together down to the Valley of the Christmas Trees.

But, ah! there is so much more to tell. The adventures of the Christmas Reindeer span many centuries, and their stories could fill countless books! Yet I must be content that at last the stories of all eight Reindeer are being shared with the world.

24

Never Say Good-Bye

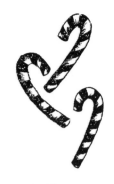

As I gathered my papers and neatly put them into folders, I surveyed my work. There were mounds of papers, notes, cassette tapes, pencils, pens, pads, and erasers. Vixen and Cupid were helping me organize everything. Donder and Dancer were quietly talking in front of Donder's fireplace.

It seemed like such a short time since I had first arrived with all of them and begun my work on these *Chronicles of the Christmas Reindeer*.

It was a quiet, peaceful evening. I was hosting our get-together tonight. Donder had helped me arrange his living room as I wished. I wanted to be able to see all of my friends as we talked. I just knew that tonight was going to be especially important to me.

As we finished sorting my papers and put the finished notes into boxes, Vixen turned to me and, trying to smile, said, "Let's go see if those cookies are ready, Lad. I really am anxious to try that famous recipe you've been raving about."

I smiled back at her and nodded, biting my lip to keep back the tears. Why was I feeling like this? I sensed that something was going to happen to me — but I had no idea what. Cupid came up and put her arm around me as we walked into the kitchen. As I took the sheet of cookies out of Donder's oven, I stumbled slightly and several cookies fell to the floor, broken. Vixen and I just stared at them for a moment, and then we all started crying. We couldn't keep pretending that nothing was wrong.

Cupid wiped her eyes and, looking at me softly, whispered, "It's not a good-bye, you know. I will never, never say good-bye, Lad."

Vixen smiled through her tears and quietly echoed this thought, "There are never any good-byes here, Lad. This will be just a short break, until you have finished what you came here to do. Then you can return to us. There's ever so much more here for you to see and wonder at—it won't seem like any time at all until you're back here where you belong: with us."

I smiled through my sadness. I had not really wanted to admit to myself that I would be going home. Even now, I didn't know exactly how long I had left to spend with the Christmas Reindeer. That's why I wanted this night to be special.

Dancer came quietly into the kitchen and stopped. Vixen and Cupid were holding me tightly, sniffling. Dancer quietly bent down to pick up the fallen cookies. He too was silently crying. I had to go back to the living room, I was so moved by their care for me.

I saw that Donder was standing in front of his bay window looking out over the snow-covered mountains. So I walked over to him and put my arm over his shoulder. He softly whispered, "I wouldn't have changed a thing, Lad."

We were standing there together when Santa and Mrs. Claus quietly let themselves in the front door. Mrs. Claus whispered, "Nicholas and Meesha picked a jewel when they chose you, Lad."

From the window, we could see Grandfather

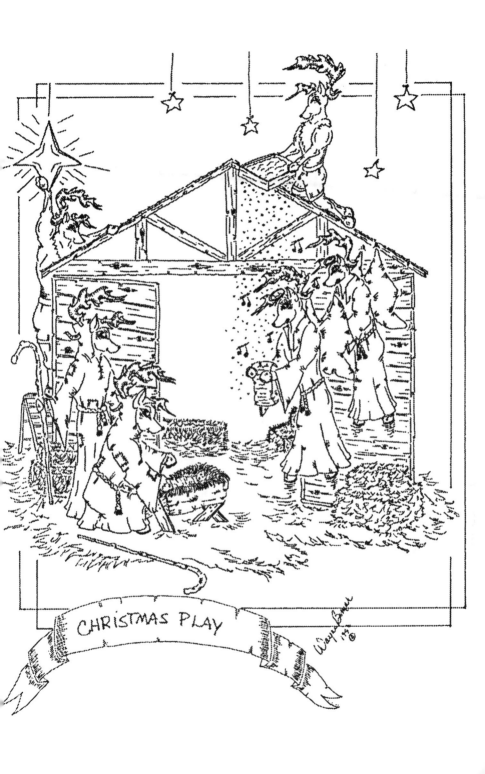

Blitzen picking his way through the fresh-fallen snow. He looked magnificent in his bright Scottish dress kilts and plaid topcoat. And he was wearing his medals of honor—every one of them.

"Meesha wanted to look special tonight," Santa whispered. "He's wearing those medals just for you, Lad."

When Blitzen entered he said, "'Tis proud I am of ye, Lad—aye, 'tis proud!"

I showed Grandfather to his chair by the fireplace. "Never forget, Lad," he said warmly, "just how much an old, old Christmas Reindeer loves ye!"

Vixen and Cupid quietly arranged the food table, though I don't think anyone felt much like eating. Since everyone had now arrived, we slowly moved around the table, filling our plates, being sociable. Yet I must have looked absolutely miserable.

After a while, Donder asked, "Grandfather, would you play for us, please?"

I saw Donder holding a set of intricately detailed bagpipes out to Grandfather Blitzen. "Yes, play Meesha! It's been so long since you've played for us," seconded Santa.

Blitzen stood up and took the bagpipes in hand. Placing the bag under his arm and adjusting the pipes over his shoulder, he looked at me and whispered, "'Tis an old, old tune I play, Lad. This is for you."

As the gentle music of the pipes drifted through the room, Santa whispered to me, "He's playing 'Mist on Loch Lomond.' It's his favorite tune. It tells of great love and joy between friends."

Although I have never experienced a walk through the heather early on a Scottish morning, or seen the Scottish highlands, I felt as though I were really *there* with Grandfather as I listened to this tune. This is how I would remember him: standing tall and proud, playing the bagpipes!

We talked long that night, all of us, of how much we loved each other, and of what a grand time we had had. I wanted to form mental pictures of each Reindeer that would carry me through the lonely times to come.

There was Cupid—gentle, little Cupid. So full of laughter and childlike innocence. Always helping, always loving and caring, wanting to please. That look of eternal wonder on her face—with soft, gentle eyes that could see straight into your heart!

Kind Vixen, who loved as a child would love: purely, simply, deeply. A big sister in her thoughtfulness, forever patting you on the shoulder or knee. Her reassuring voice that was like the whisper of the gentle wind.

And Comet, the forever teenager. So full of energy, so full of love. I thought of the looks of puzzlement that would flash from his sky-blue eyes, as he took in everything around him at once. Comet, ever ready to fly through time if but one child needed him.

Then there was Prancer, who would knot up his brow and look worried, but could melt at another's need. He contributed his hurried pace when help was needed. And he constantly kept watch on his cousin, Dancer. I sensed his immense love for us all.

Then, of course, that trickster Dancer, with his sparkling green eyes! The way he would cock one eyebrow up when he was ready to pull a prank on someone. His high, shrill laugh when he thought he had gotten away with something. The way he would look at Blitzen with his head down and antlers drooping as the older Reindeer would scold him. Yet the way he brightened when Grandfather told him all was well. Dancer, "Magical Laughter."

Dasher, gullible Dasher, the brunt of Dancer's practical jokes—at least until I came! Dasher's soft, hazel eyes with that "tell me, I'll believe it" quality. The way he would rip open a gift, like a child, with squeals and shouts of delight. And how he would cry unashamedly as Vixen dried his tears.

The mental picture I had of my friend Donder would fill a book. He was and still is a true brother to me. Explaining things, helping, reassuring me that he would take care of everything. How the others would come to him and to Blitzen for advice and help. He would answer to any need at the drop of a Christmas hat. His strength would flow into you when you needed him. He was the eternal big brother to be there to protect you and guide you.

As I looked at Donder across the room talking with Blitzen, I could feel his self-confidence and self-assurance flowing through the room, covering us all like a warm, comforting blanket. I wondered, when he became as old as Blitzen, would he too be honored with the name "Grandfather?"

Donder. The "Stout Puller of Faith." I thought of him a thousand years from now, flying high through cold, clear skies on Christmas Eve, pulling the great sleigh full of happiness. *Would he remember me?*

He looked straight across the room at me, right into my eyes, and I knew the answer was Yes!

Then my thoughts turned to Blitzen—Meesha, "Forever Wisdom and Strength." The twinkling firelight glittered in sparkling reflections against his great antlers—which he held high and proud. Stardust

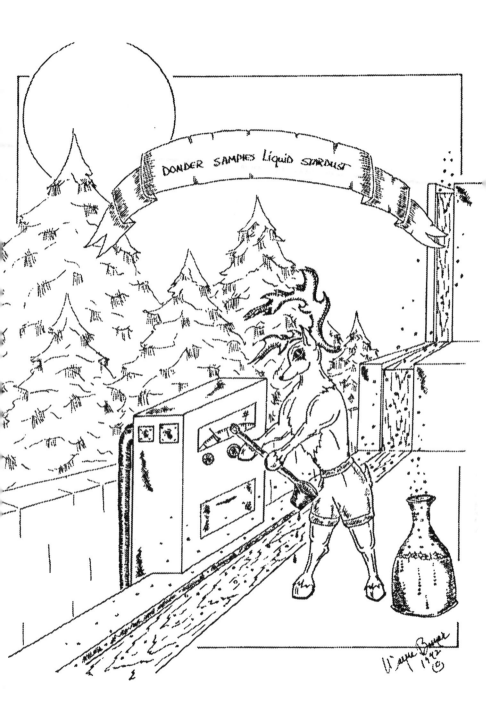

shimmered through them. Blitzen, the oldest and first-chosen Christmas Reindeer! Wisest of them all. By himself, he had captured the secrets of the stars and had flown the timeless wind-currents of Christmas. The centuries were etched on his face. His gray whiskers sparkled with age and time. How very proud Grandfather is. He is with all of them... a part of them. He would always know what to do. He would always be there for them and for the children of the world, throughout time.

I would always picture Grandfather Blitzen in his splendid Scottish kilts, silhouetted against a sparkling, moonlit sky, his head held high, playing the bagpipes. I would forever hear the soft music of the pipes wafting through my heart. And I would think often of the Grandfather... the first Christmas Reindeer.

25

With Love, From All of Us

I slowly opened my eyes. I felt strangely disoriented—even a little chilled as I lay there in bed. I supposed that Donder had carried me into my room, as he had done before when I'd fallen asleep in an easy chair or at my desk.

As I gradually wakened, and my eyes adjusted to the light, I thought about the night before. What a wonderful time I had had just being with all of the Christmas Reindeer. I would have to thank Vixen and Cupid today for helping me in the kitchen last night with the cookies.

Slowly, I pulled the covers off. I remember thinking that I had to go down to the North Pole laundry today, since the sheets smelled somewhat musty. I couldn't imagine why, as we had washed them two days earlier. Oh, well… Maybe Dasher and Comet would be there, and we could just sit and talk again. That was always fun.

I yawned and swung my feet over the edge of the bed, and stood up, stretching. Suddenly, in mid-stretch, my eyes popped wide open! I quickly looked around the room. *This wasn't Donder's house!* Where a window should have been, there wasn't one. There was no garland hanging from the ceiling. No Christmas ornaments over the doorway. No smell of holly and evergreen everywhere...

"Donder!!!" I screamed, running from the room. I ran through this strange place that I didn't recognize. From room to room I went, screaming for Donder. I heard only the sound of the echo of my own voice. I became scared. "Donder, where are you?"

My arms fell to my side and I slumped down in a dusty chair. I gazed around this room and realized... I was home. In my own house. I sat there for about an hour, I suppose, not moving.

My tears spattered the thick dust that covered the floor. Finally I got up and went back to my bedroom. My feet made small clouds of dust as I walked. I sat down on the bed and pondered it all. "It was a dream," I thought. "All of it was but a dream. I am home. I've always been home."

Everywhere, familiar things stared back at me. The house certainly was in a state of neglect. As I reached for a broom, I remembered how wonderful the dream had been—and how real it had seemed.

I decided to go clean the living room first.

As I walked down the hall, I paused in front of a large mirror I had hanging on the wall. Then I saw something, just out of the corner of my eye. It was my *hair!* There was something in my hair. I put my hand up to my head, and, pulling it back, saw that some kind of sparkly substance was on my hand. It twinkled merrily as I held it to my eyes for a closer look. "What in the world have I slept on?" I wondered. I shook my head and saw even more of the particles falling. Abruptly I sat down on the floor, my eyes wide open.

Something clicked. I quickly jumped up and ran to my bedroom, looking frantically for something. There it was, on my dresser—a big, red envelope! And I knew I hadn't put it there.

Snatching it up, I tore the envelope open and saw even more sparkles fall to the floor. My hands trembled as I read, "If 'tis a smile ye seek, give a gift. If 'tis love and happiness ye seek, give of yourself." Even before the letter touched the floor, where I had dropped it, I was running down the hall, toward my living room, crying.

In front of the closed double doors, in the thick dust that covered the floor, were some unusual prints. I recognized those hoofprints! I grabbed the doorknobs and threw open the doors to my living room, and was immediately enveloped by a nearly blinding light. When my eyes finally adjusted to the light, I gazed around the room.

There was the desk I had worked on, my typewriter sitting on top of it. My papers, notes, cassettes... everything! The room was now alive with Christmas! Living greens hung from the ceilings. The odor of holly and evergreen filled my nostrils. I ran into the middle of the room and spun myself around, hugging myself tightly in my joy!

I scampered from treasure to treasure, touching everything and crying aloud. Hanging from my walls were pictures of all the Christmas Reindeer. Just over my fireplace was a portrait of Santa Claus with his arm around—me! That picture, I remembered now, had been taken in the Great Hall of Toys not a week ago! Sitting beside my typewriter was the picture of Donder and me, signed: "To You, From Me. Your Pal, Donder." My sweater with Comet's portrait on it was hanging over a chair—the chair that Donder had made especially for me. It sparkled with stardust.

I next saw an enormous bowl of chip wafers, still warm, sitting on top of a table that I recognized instantly. It was the first Christmas sled that Grandfather Blitzen had had sitting in front of his fireplace!

There were letters from all of them hanging from an enormous Christmas tree that I knew to be Grandfather Blitzen's. Plucking the letters from the tree, I read each one. They all said in different ways, "We love you, Lad, we love you. Finish your work and come quickly home to us. Merry Christmas!"

I cried with joy and swayed to and fro. *It wasn't a dream! I had really been there! I had really been there!*

The entire room twinkled with stardust. I could almost see the Christmas Reindeer standing beside me, laughing and smiling—now that I had all these precious memories of our time together. Each treasure brought back a memory so vivid, I felt like I was still there... with them. I would hurry with my work. I would finish! They were all waiting for me to return to them—to come *home!*

From across the room, my typewriter sparkled and glimmered as I had never seen it do before. I walked over to it, and, bending down, saw the reason for such a sparkle of luster. Picking up the gold chain, I held the medallion that hung from it close to my eyes and read: "Meesha, Forever Wisdom and Strength."

I quickly placed the chain with the medallion around my neck and sat down at my typewriter.

The sudden ringing of the phone shattered my train of thought. Looking just behind the typewriter, I saw a sparkling red telephone! It had no cords going to it or coming from it, yet it continued to ring!

I picked up the receiver, grinning. A most familiar voice came laughing out of the receiver: "Hey, Lad... it's Donder!"

I burst out laughing and crying at once.

"I have some great news, Lad," he said excitedly. "Santa and Grandfather Blitzen have granted me a leave of absence. I thought I might come down to be with you for a couple of months. Kind of help you get the place cleaned of cobwebs. You know, you were gone almost a year. The place was sure a mess when we brought you home last night! Maybe I could help you get organized and keep you company."

I could hardly talk, I was so happy just to hear Donder's voice again. I choked back my tears and stuttered into the phone, "I'll put on the water for hot chocolate right now!"

"Great!!! See you in about three hours," he answered. "Hey, Lad, everyone sends their love," he whispered.

I gently put the receiver back on the phone. After drying my eyes, I placed a sheet of paper in the typewriter roller and typed:

Chapter 1:

The Journey Begins— Christmas Eve Magic

Christmas Eve—1968—and now, as I write...

Coming soon!
Further Adventures of the Christmas Reindeer! Volume II

About the Author

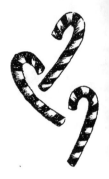

Wayne Bomar has made a commitment to bring back the magic of Christmas. He is a man who truly believes in the sirit of the season and is working to help us all recapture those precious, wonderful days of our childhood.

Wayne Bomar is a native Tennessean who lives in Gallatin, Tennessee. He has served 25 years as Tennessee State Park Lt. Ranger and Park Superintendent. In 1989, he promised Santa and Mrs. Claus that the lives and adventures of the immortal Christmas Reindeer would be told to the world. In this book he tells of the love and dedication the Christmas Reindeer carry in their hearts for the people of the entire world. This book describes the "home of Santa Claus and the Christmas Reindeer at the top of the world, just under the great stor of the North—a magical, wondrous place where wishes are granted and dreams do come true."